Traditional Styles of Yogic Science
Understanding Traditional Ways of Performing Yoga

Dr. VINEET KUMAR SHARMA

Dr. SUNIL DESHMUKH

ISBN: 172122078X
ISBN-13: 978-1721220786

Dedicated to my parents

(Equivalent to God for me)

&

Brothers

(Strong ends besides me)

&

Yoga Lovers

ABOUT THIS BOOK

To clarify and expand your horizon to the entire, wonderful world of Yoga, this text has been developed. It is helpful for the students of yogic sciences at the college and university level and also for those who have keen interest to learn and understand the various traditional styles of yogic science. The entire material deals with the history, origin and different styles of yoga like **Bhakti Yoga, Jnana Yoga, Karma Yoga, Raja Yoga, Hatha Yoga, Dhyan Yoga, Mantra Yoga, Kundalini Yoga.** *The author keeps the simple and easiest explanations of Sanskrit Surtas of traditional yogic literature about various styles of yoga for better understanding which is the main difficulty faced by the students at graduate and post graduate level.*

This book consist the 10 chapters, starting with the chapter which discusses the Introduction of Yoga, Historical Development of Yoga in Veda, Upnishad, Purana, Ramayana, Mahabharat and in Shreemad Bhagwat Gita. Readers will get the connectivity in each part of this book that may help them to maintain the flow of reading. Further, in following chapters the various traditional and ancient styles of yoga has been discussed in the connection with ancient literature.

We hope that this book will serve the purpose of better understanding of yoga and its traditional styles. The readers are requested to send their feedback and suggestions about the book or about the problems which they encounter, directly to the authors for further improvement in the text. You may reach them through;

Dr. V.K. Sharma #sharmavineet654@gmail.com
Dr. Sunil Deshmukh ##sunildeshmukhlnipe@gmail.com

ACKNOWLEDGMENTS

I would like to express my gratitude to Dr. Sunil Deshmukh (Co-Author) for his effort to make this work successful by giving technical support and being a kind thoughtful inspiration. Your advices to prepare the content in easy form are priceless.

I would also like to express my special appreciation and thanks to my Ph.D. supervisor Professor (Dr.) Jayashree Acharya. You have been a tremendous mentor, teacher and role model for me. I would like to thank you for encouraging me for this work. Your guidance is priceless. I would also like to thank my teacher Dr. Nibu R. Krishna, for helping in and beyond the scope of this work in life.

A special thanks to my family. Words cannot express how grateful I am to my parents for all the sacrifices that you've made on my behalf. Your prayer for me was what sustained me thus for.

In the end I would like to thank the almighty lord for helping me find my path and passion in life.

CONTENTS

CHAPTER-1

INTRODUCTION OF YOGA

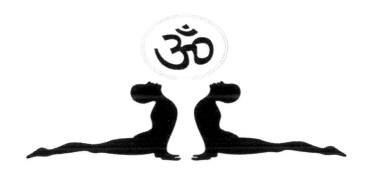

Figure no. 1 Yogic Practice [1]

"Yoga began with the first person wanting to be healthy and happy all the time."

(Sri Swami Satchidananda, 1970)

"Everyone has in him something divine, something his own, a chance of perfection and strength in however small a sphere which God offers him to take or refuse. The task is to find it, develop it & use it. The chief aim of education should be to help the growing soul to draw out that in itself which is best and make it perfect for a noble use."

(Sir Aurobindo, 1995)

---

[1] Retrieved on 02.11.2014 [http://yogahousestroudsburg.com/wp-content/uploads/2011/12/8.jpg]

"Yoga is a light, which once lit, will never dim; the better your practice, the brighter the flame."

(B.K.S. Iyengar, 2014)

"Yoga, an ancient but perfect science, deals with the evolution of humanity. This evolution includes all aspects of one's being, from bodily health to self-realization. Yoga means union - the union of body with consciousness and consciousness with the soul. Yoga cultivates the ways of maintaining a balanced attitude in day to day life and endows skill in the performance of one's actions."

(B.K.S. Iyengar, 2001)

Yoga, the discipline of right living and is proposed to be merged in day-to-day life. It can be applied on all facets of the individual: the vital, physical, intellectual, psychic, emotional and spiritual (Rama, 2002).

Yoga is a science of right living and it work when integrated in our daily life. It works on all aspects of the person-the physical, mental, emotional, and psychic and spirituals. Generally the word 'Yoga' means 'Union'. Etymologically it has been derived from Sanskrit root 'Yuj' which means to bind, join attach or yoke. Yoga signifies communion of self with the supreme universal spirit to obtain relief from pain and suffering. According to Panini grammar it has three meanings- Union (Yujir Yoge), Samadhi (Yug Samadhau) and constraint, restraint (Yug Samyamane). Examples for these usages can be found in the sacred and classical Sanskrit Literature.

2

Yoga standing for mental concentration is the theme of the entire Indian systems dealing with Yoga. Therefore the second deviation of the word Yoga consists in the stopping or blocking the activities of the mind. According to Bhagvat Gita, perfection in action is known as Yoga.

There are too many misconceptions clouding the science of Yoga. People perceive it to be some kind of black or white magic, sorcery, physical or mental debauchery through which miraculous feats can be performed. For some it is an extremely dangerous practice which should be limited to only those who have renounced the world. Few others think it to be a kind of mental and physical acrobatics that is compatible only to a Hindu mind.[2]

---

[2] Retrieved on 02.10.2014 [http://www.swamil.com/history-yoga.htm]

CHAPTER - 2

HISTORICAL DEVELOPMENT OF YOGA

YOGA IN VEDA-S

Modern is indebted to ancient India for its precious gift of ideology and technology of Yoga. The seeds of Yoga systems may be discovered in the Vedic Samhitas because Veda-s is the foundation of Indian culture philosophy and religion. The Veda-s has been generally interpreted as the basis of ritualistic traditions of Indian, but the spiritual elements are also profusely available in the Vedic hyms. Hiranyagarbha of the earliest Vedic and Upishads lore is spoken of as the first being of reveal Yoga.[3]

Rigveda is the oldest and the most important among the four Vedas. For the derivation of the words "Yoga", the vedic line yujyate amina iti Yogah or vehicle to achieve some desired aim or object. The Rigveda samhita advises us to unite our mind through the process of Yoga with Brahman, the Absolute Being.

Here again in Rigveda, it is mentioned that a person follows the path Yoga for gaining control over mind senses. In this the Yunjate again gives the idea of Yoga and is related to Manas or mind. This not only to unite the mind with the self but also to unite senses, which refers mental as well as physical Yoga.

---

[3] Retrieved on 02.10.2014 [http://www.swamil.com/history-yoga.htm]

In Yajurveda, some references directly or indirectly to yogic system can be adducted. The same reference "yujyate mama...." of Rigveda is repeated in the Yajurveda for the sake of putting emphasis on the mental Yoga.

Further the last mantra of the Yajurveda symbolically says, "The face of truth is cover by a golden lid "which in the sun, "I am that I am"

The first two sentences of this mantra have been separated with some addition in the Upnishad, these two mantras say that "The face of Truth is covered by the golden lid."O! Puskar, remove this lid for the realization of Truth.

In Samveda, it is concerned, with the exception of some mantras; its basic quality is that its mantras are musical in its nature. When the mantras are sung musically, they are called samans. If me say that music helps to concentrate the mind, all its mantras are helpful for mental concentration. But the seeds of Yoga systems are not directly observable in this samhita.

The Artharvaveda is most important for the study of yoga practices .Some of the mantras of this Veda refer to some of the aspects of Yoga system. They lay emphasis on the vital energy working within the individual as well as in the whole universe. A complete hymm containing 26 verses is devoted to the description of the Brahma.[4]

---

[4] Retrieved on 02.10.2014 [http://www.abc-of-yoga.com/beginnersguide/yogahistory.asp]

YOGA IN UPNISHAD-S

Next to vedas the Upanishad-s are more important repositories of vedic thought. They have inspired the people to gain spiritual knowledge. The Upanished represent the body of the spiritual realisations based upon individual experience. The quest of Upinashads is truth and this quest is more through realisation than through intellect. Truth is self-luminous. The invocation of Isavasya Upanishad is of the paramount important. It strikes the key notes of the whole Upnishad teaching. It contains the crux of the Vedic thought in all its purity and simplicity.

The Prasnaupanishad describes the superiority of the prana to all other senses including the manas. It is said that the whole universe remains under the control of prana.

In the Mundakaupanishad, it is also advised that one should meditate on the self in the form of Om.

In the Chandogyaupanishad, there is a detailed discussion regarding the spiritual elements within our organism and in the whole universe. The dialogue takes place between Narad and Sanat Kurma who explains the significance of Citta to Narad. Since Chitta is the abode of all types of thinking and control over the Citta is essential for the flower of the path of Yoga. After having followed the significance of Citta, Narad asks Sanat Kurma if there was anything more significant than Citta.

YOGA IN PURANA-S

The Puranas forms a vast literature of Hinduism.
Among the available Puranas eighteen are important. Out
of these few Puranas give details about Yoga. The Puranas
are many but the one that is most important as a
background of a definite spirituality and constructive
philosophy is Bhagavata Purana. The Bhagvata Purana
explains Bhakti Yoga. Linga Purana gives the details about
Yama, Niyama and Pranayam. Vayu purana gives details
about Pratyahara, Dharana and Dhyana.

The Bhagavata indeed opens with the fine emphasis
upon transcendent Truth from which emerges the life of
shadows. Devotion to lord is also a form of Yoga because
the recitation of The Devine name also helps to concentrate
the mind. The Bhakti Yoga and the other forms of Yoga are
also described in details in all the Purana in general and in
the Bhagvat Purana. Through the Bhakti Yoga one can
attain the Grace of God whether that God is qualified or
non-qualified.[5]

YOGA IN EPICS

THE RAMAYANA: The Ramayana consists of 24,000
shlokas distributed among seven chapters. The great book
of Yoga known as Yoga Vasistha was written in this time
Ramayana. Valmiki wrote his magnum opus in the ideal
ornate giving a silent touch of transformation to the
feelings. The Ramayana, more than any other scriptures,

---

[5] Retrieved on 02.10.2014 [http://www.gofc.org/history_of_yoga.html]

has been able to maintain freshness of appeal for Dharma. It has done the noble task of raising the nation - wide spiritual tone of society. It is rich in Vedic values. Valmiki's theme in The Ramayan remains human with a concept of character in which virtues of truth, honour, charity, duty and self-restraint illumine every trying moment and impending doom in the minds of people. In the great time of Yoga Tulsi Das's Bhakti Yoga the same three means (devotion, love and surrender) or mind and self-realization. Consistency of effort is essential in Yoga-Sadhana. Continuous toil with strong interest is considered to be very important and helpful for an early success in attainment of the Chief Goal, Patanjali, in the great Sage has said.[6]

THE MAHABHARAT: The Mahabharata has been declared as the treasure knowledge. Its author himself says that whatever is not here is no-where. According to Mahabharata it assumed that the system of Yoga started from Brahma himself. His son Vaisistha was called so because he had controlled his mind and mastered his sense. Without sense control, Yoga is not possible. Self-controlled has been described in The Mahabharata as the highest duty for the wise persons and the man of tapas.

---

[6] Retrieved on 02.10.2014 [http://yoga.ygoy.com/2010/05/22/the-history-yoga-preclassical-yoga/]

YOGA IN SHREEMAD BHAGAVAT GITA

The book that has been and still the main spring in Hindu's life is The Gita, as the part of The Mahabharata, and has been treated as a separate book of Indian spirituality. It generally said that the Upanishads are the Cows, the milkman is Krishna and milk is The Gita. The Bhagavat Gita is known as a jewel of Mahabharata gives the definition of Yoga. All the 18 chapters in The Gita are designated as types of Yoga to train the body and mind. The 18 chapters are reduced into 4 chapters-The Karma Yoga, The Raja Yoga, The Bhakti Yoga and The Jnana Yoga. Traditions told that spiritual life begins with Karma Yoga, perfection in action. But the action is the duty of man.

The Karma Yoga of the Gita is a unique philosophy of action and it declares the nature has given the right of action to man only and the right of the result of action is under authority of nature.[7]

---

[7] Retrieved on 02.10.2014
[http://www.clivir.com/lessons/show/history-of-yoga-classification-of-yoga-history-into-four-periods.html]

CHAPTER - 3

BHAKTI YOGA

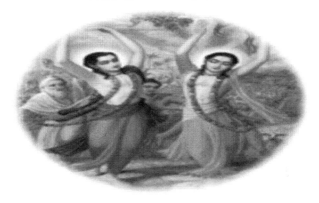

Figure No. 2 Bhakti Yoga [8]

Bhakti Yoga is the easiest and natural way for God – realization. It is deeply concerned with our life. This path of devotion is for everyone. Anybody can practice it. Even the vilest man can start and gradually improvement will take place. [9]

The Narada Bhakti Sutra defines Bhakti in the second verse as follows:

Sa Tvasmin Parama-premarupa://

---Narada Bhakti Sutras 1/2

---

[8] Retrieved on 04.10.2014
[http://www.umich.edu/~bhakti/Bhakti_Yoga_Society_@_Univ._of_Michigan!/Bhakti_Yoga_Society_files/droppedImage_1.jpg]
[9] Retrieved on 04.10.2014
[http://www.venkatesaya.com/512.sutras/narada.php?p=01_02&menuid=2]

Means: Bhakti is the supreme love for Him (God). The object of real devotion is only God and nothing else. This love should be pure and powerful; there should not be any kind of selfish idea associated with it. Therefore one should not expect anything like wealth, prosperity or any worldly object from God – not even the happiness.[10]

The Bhagwad Gita discusses the Bhakti Yoga as an easier path of Yoga. The Gita says that when a devotee's love for God reaches its climax, his love for God is known as the Yoga of devotion. The devotee wants nothing return; and when he loves God in such a way his love takes the form of Yoga which is called the Yoga of devotion or Bhakti Yoga.

In the twenty second verse of the eighth chapter Lord Krishna reflects the Yoga of devotion when he says:

**Purusah Sa Parah Parth Bhaktya Lavhyastbananya /
Yasyantahsthani bhutani Yena Sarvamidam Taam //**

Meaning: O' Arjuna, that eternal unmanifest supreme Purusa in whom all beings reside and by whom all this is pervaded is attainable only through exclusive Devotion.

The twenty sixth verse of the ninth chapter highlights how a devotee with his pure love wins the heart of the Lord:

---

[10] K. Kumar; (2009), *Super Science of Yoga,* p.p. 124-130, Standard Publishers (India) New Delhi

**Patram Puspam Phalam Toyam Yo me Bhaktya Prayacchati /
Tadaham Bhaktyupachrtmasnami Prayatatmanah //**

Meaning: who so ever offers to me with love a leaf, a flower, a fruit or even water; I appear in person before that disinterested devotee of sinless mind and delightfully partake of that article offered by him with love.

When we go through the seventeenth verse of the twelfth chapter we find what lord Krishna Himself explains devotion as:

**Yo Na Hrsyati Na Dvesti Na Sochati Na Kanksati/
Subhasubha Parityagi Bhaktimanyah SA Me Priyah//**

Meaning: He who neither rejoices nor hates, nor grieves, nor desires and who renounces both good and evil actions and is full of devotion, is dear to me;

The final aim of Bhakti is the communion of individual consciousness with supreme or Universal consciousness. But before we come to this stage, there are different stages of Bhakti which act at the deeper level of mind to transform the mental structure, the mental conditioning. Goswami Tulsi Das explains the nine steps of Bhakti in Sri Ram Carita Manasa (Ramayana) in a very specific form as:

**Navadha Bhagati Kahaun Tohi Pahin /
Savadhan Sunu Dharu Mana Mahin //
Pratham Bhagati Santanh Kar Sanga /
Dusari Rati Mam Katha Prasanga //**

Meaning: Satsanga (associate with truth or the company of truthful person) is considered to be the first form of Bhakti. Being near a saint and having their Satsanga, instruction and guidance can be one form of Bhakti. Another form of the same Bhakti can be taken as analysing the Truth and spiritual life; but whatever it is the main emphasis is on one's being in the company of truth. Now, if we also define this psychologically, the Truth here represents a quality which is gained after attaining discernment. If there is no discernment Truth one needs to have the power, the force of discrimination.

One can attain this form of Bhakti through Sadhana, whether that Sadhana is being in the company of a person who is enlightened, absorbing his or her vibrations and allowing the inner mind to experience it, or whether that Sadhana is self-analysis, trying to develop the faculty of discernment through a meditative process or whether that Sadhana is self-analysis, trying to develop the faculty of discernment through a meditative process or way of life. According to their level of life and consciousness, everyone has to give their own definition to Satsanga, or being in the company of Truth.

The second form of Bhakti is Katha Prasanga, in colloquial language listening to Lilas or story of divine beings. These Lilas about enlightened beings can help inspire us to accept a different lifestyle, mentality and mode of behaviour. However, it also has a psychological meaning. It is the nature of the mind to involve itself in constant gossip and criticism. The moment one stops the mind gossiping and criticizing, it becomes calm, peaceful and fixed, and it begins to experience a different kind of senses and objects. That is the experience of Sunyata, the void, awareness of a different quality manifesting:

**Gur Pad Pankaj Seva Tisari Bhagati Aman /
Chauthi Bhagati Mam Gun Gan Karai Kapat Taji Gan //**

Meaning: The third form of Bhakti is Aman, becoming egoless it is necessary to have Vairgya and live in the world, but not be of the world. In fact, the entire philosophy of the Bhagwad Gita is based on this very principle – one should do his own work, should perform own Dharma, carry out all obligations, but should not think that he is the indispensable one. One should not have any attachment. One may be attached to something, whether to a person, or to the results of an action. Wherever there is even the slightest inkling of attachment, there is a connection with ego, possessiveness, desire, ambition are all involved in attachment. To be egoless is to give a different vision of life where we are able to experience the state of non-being.

The fourth form of Bhakti is Japa. Japa literarily means continuous repetition of a Mantra or God's name. it is constant remembrance that, who lives in this body, the individual self and the cosmic self which pervades the entire universe ,are one. In Japa, the essence has to be realized. A raindrop and water in the river or ocean are two different things, but they are composed of the same essence or matter. Japa is the process of identifying with the Divine or cosmic nature. It is a method by which a person who has attained Viveka and Vairagya can disassociate the individual self-form the manifest dimension and link with the cosmic dimension:

Mantra Jap Mam Drirh Biswasa /
Pancham Bhajan So Bed Prakasa //

Meaning: The fifth form of bhakti is Bhajana-incorporating the transcendental, humanitarian and unconditioned qualities into everyday life. The qualities which we express in our lives are conditioned qualities which gave some restrictions and motivation in them. The real language of living is expressing these qualities which are cosmic, divine and human, which are not conditioned, but which are free from every kind of mental or manifest impression. When one is free from the attractions and repulsions of life, love is experienced .So, removing the conditions which we create in the expression of a quality is the fifth form of Bhakti:

Chhath Dam Sil Birali Bahu Karma/
Nirat Nirantar Sajjan Dharma//
Satavam Sam Modi Maya Jag Dekha/
Moten Sant Adhika Kari Leka//

Meaning: The sixth form of Bhakti is Total involvement in Sajjan Dharma, i.e. manifesting in one's life the qualities which are divine and human while following one's dharma. Generally, when we live a quality in our life, we tend to isolate ourselves from the dharma belonging to the realm of the body, the realm of the mind and emotions, and also from the dharma governing the spiritual dimension. It sounds easy, but we find it very difficult to combine the principles of spirituality and awareness with the normal, external environment and life style. Instead of feeling the rejection and repulsion inside, instead of identifying with a personal desire, live life from moment to moment by accepting situations as they come up, and follow dharma accordingly.

The seventh form of Bhakti is seeing the spark of life and divinity in each every one. There should be no distinction between one and another. There should be no concept of high and low, but there is identification. Seeing the divinity within self as well as other beings; whether animate or inanimate, is the highest form of compassion where the individual self is totally eradicated (Kaput):

**Athavam Jalathabh Santosa /
Sapnehun Nahin Dekhai Pardosa //
Navam Saral Sab San Chhalahina /
Mam Bharosa Hiyan Harasa Na Dina //**

Meaning: The eighth form of Bhakti is contentment, not seeing fault in other beings. One who does not struggle, or fight. Who does not see any kind of fault in other people, but who lives and flows with life, is content. If there is acceptance of the natural law, to develop the acceptance is one of the important forms of Bhakti.

The ninth form of Bhakti is Atma nivedana – total surrender, total fusion or total merger. Atma means self and nivedana means to offer. It happens when even the last vestige of individual identify is dissolved in cosmic awareness. At that of Atma Nivedana is not very easy to attain. If faith becomes powerful and takes that real experience where the existence ceased to this world this will be the state of Atma Nivedana:

Nav Mahun Ekau Jinh Ken Hoi /
Nari Purusa Sacharachar Koi //

Meaning: The ninth forms of Bhakti is not only for the fulfilment of only the requirement but these can lead to discrimination and ultimately the final state i.e. Samadhi the goal of Yoga.

Bhakti is of two types: Para and Apara. As we go on, in the preparatory stage, we unavoidably stand in need of many concrete helps to enables us to get on and indeed the mythological and symbolical parts of all religions.

When Bhakti has reached its peaks, it is called the Para, no more is there any fear of hideous manifestations of fanaticism. In the words of Swami Vivekananda: The one great advantage of Bhakti is that it is the easiest and the most natural way to reach the great divine.

Significance of Bhakti Yoga

Unwavering Devotion & Love for God

Bhakti, according to the Gita, is the love for God and love reinforced by a true knowledge of the glory of God. It surpasses the love for all things worldly. This love is constant and is centred in God and God alone, and cannot be shaken under any circumstances whether in prosperity or in adversity.[11]

- The ideal devotee (Bhakta) does not hate any living being.
- The ideal devotee cultivates friendship and compassion.
- The ideal devotee gives up the feeling of "I and Mine".
- The ideal devotee be unmoved by happiness or misery.
- The ideal devotee is forgiving.
- The ideal devotee strives for self-control.
- The ideal devotee always is content with what he/she has.
- The ideal devotee has a strong determination.
- The ideal devotee surrenders his/her mind and intellect to God.
- The ideal devotee not afraid of anyone; and none in the world should fear him/her.
- The ideal devotee desires nothing.
- The ideal devotee is pure and efficient.
- The ideal devotee is free from elation, anger, fear and turbulence of mind.
- The ideal devotee is indifferent to what befalls him/her.

---

[11] Retrieved on 04.10.2014
[http://hinduism.about.com/od/thegita/a/gitabhakti.htm]

- The ideal devotee is free from weakness of mind.[12]
- The ideal devotee free from the feeling that he/she is an independent agent.
- The ideal devotee does not have any feeling of elation and enmity or desire.
- The ideal devotee develops an attitude of mind which rejects good as well as bad things.
- The ideal devotee does not have attachments and should accept pain and pleasure, honour and disgrace, heat and cold equally as his/her portion.
- The ideal devotee looks upon friends and foes alike.
- The ideal devotee not indulge in idle talk.
- The ideal devotee not attached to any fixed abode.
- The ideal devotee is steadfast in mind.[13]

---

[12] Retrieved on 04.10.2014
[http://www.yogamag.net/archives/1992/djuly92/bhkyog.shtml]
[13] ibid www.yogamag.net

CHAPTER - 4

JANANA YOGA

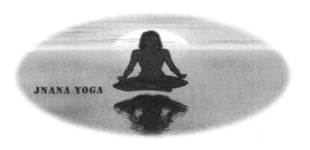

Figure No. 3 Jnana Yoga [14]

The word Jnana literary means knowledge and wisdom, thus it is known as Yoga of Knowledge and wisdom. What is that knowledge? It is understanding or experience of the self. To know the self through knowledge or wisdom is Jnana Yoga.

This path of yoga deals directly with the highest of all human desires – the desire to know the Truth – and it gives an explanation of what Truth means and shows the practical way of realizing it. Truth is that which is not subject to change, death, decay and destruction. It never changes at any time; it was never born, and will never die. It is self-existent and does not depend on anything. Gyana Yoga is the science that provides a systematized and organized method of study in order to fulfil this desire to

---

[14] Retrieved on 04.10.2014
[http://www.umich.edu/~bhakti/Bhakti_Yoga_Society_@_Univ._of_M ichigan!/Bhakti_Yoga_Society_files/droppedImage_1.jpg]

know the Truth The truth or reality is only Atman the knowledge of self, which is ultimate. To know that and to know the importance of that Atman Lord Krishna says in The Gita:[15]

**Na Jayate Mriyate Va Kadachinnayam Bhutva Bhavita Van A Bhuyah /
Ajo Nityah Saswatoayam Purano Na Hanyate
Hanyamane Sarire //**

- **Srimadbhagvad Gita 2/20**

Meaning: This is never born, nor does it die. This is unborn, eternal, and changeless ever-itself. It is not killed when the body dies. All these specialization is of the atman (soul) only.

When the aspirant becomes aware of this ultimate truth he starts realizing the self and start following the path of jnan yoga and ultimately gets liberated from all worldly bondage of karma. in this sense lord krisna again says in Gita that :

**Kanmajam Buddhiyaukta Hi Phalam Tyaktya
Manisinab/
Janmahandhavinirmukatab Padam Gachchan
Tyaanamayam//**

- **Srimadhbhagvad Gita 2/51**

Meaning: The aspirant of jnan yoga after knowing the ultimate truth possessed of this evenness of mind and

15 K. Kumar; (2009), *Super Science of Yoga,* p.p. 131-135, Standard Publishers (India) New Delhi

abandoning the fruits of their actions feed for ever from the fetters o birth and go to that state which is beyond all evil that is moksa.

Hence all the Sadhana in which intellect of knowledge is used as object is Jnana yoga: as the holy Gita describes Jnana yoga with the name of Samkhya yoga, but basically the Sadhana of Vedanta is known as Jnana yoga. Since in Vedanta the knowledge is the main path of yoga; through which the aspirant become one with brahma.

According to the principle of Jnana yoga the atman is Ananda Svarupa (as blissful), Jnanuwarupa (knowledge form) Sat (truth), Nitya (forever), Suddha (pure) and Buddha (intellect). In the real sense the atman is brahma it-self. Only Brahman is the reality, there is no existence except it.

Brahman is self-focused, endless, uninterrupted, unborn, conscious and blissful; As the fire is one and reflects in different form in several places, the same is the case with Brahman, it is one bur appears in the form of soul of every creatures and it is beyond all of them.

According to Jnana yoga the knowledge of unity of Jiva (the individual being) and Brahman (The Supreme Being). Bring the aspirants to the state of Moksa, the liberation. In other words the knowledge of Brahman and liberation from all the worries is Moksa itself. According to this tradition it is possible only when the oneness of Jiva and Brahman has been proved, it has been said that the aspirant of higher level becomes able to know that reality only through listening the Srutivakya (the sayings of

Brahman). He becomes able to remove the difference between Jiva and Brahman. According to Vedanta this reality is possible only through knowledge.

The practice of Jnana yoga is divided into two paths: Antaranga practice and Bahiranga practice. Bahiranga (external) practice includes Viveka, Vairagara, Satsamti and Mumuksurva: whereas the Antarnga (internal) practice includes Sranvana Manana and Nidhidyasana.

Viveka (discrimination): The practitioner has to develop and cultivate the ability to recognize what is impermanent, temporary and fleeting in life as the Sadhaka experiences the fact-what is of everlasting value and pointing to the eternal. The practitioner becomes able to discriminate the superficial and the essential; as well as the illusory reality on the surface and the absolute reality in the inner, deep dimension of existence. In this way the person tries to scrutinize analyses and evaluate constantly the experiences, inclinations, decisions and actions.

Vairagaya (dispassion): In the practice of Varigaya the practitioner has to guard his mind against becoming possessed, infatuated and even slightly disturbances like attachment to things that bring sensual satisfaction. The opposite of Vairagaya is raga (passion) which means originally colouring, which indicates that passions are, in fact obstructions of the mind which do not allow clear vision. To achieve the clarity of mind (which is essential for final knowledge and wisdom) attachments and passions must he avoided and abolished.

Satsampati (six-attainments): This discipline includes a six fold instruction of self-education for success on the path of yoga which are as follows:

- Sama: The cultivation of tranquility of the mind.
- Dama: Self-control in action
- Uparati: Means eradicating the eagerness to possess.
- Titiksa: To have patience
- Sraddha: Confidence (in the meaning of faith).
- Samadhana: Intentness of the mind

Mumuksutva (longing for liberation): This fourth Sadhana of Vedanta is very important. It should be understood as the intense desire to get the higher level of consciousness i.e. Samadhi. The Sadhaka or aspirant should develop a positive desire for liberation. Its development is supported by the previous endeavours as the advanced ability to discriminate the unsatisfactory superficial reality and the safety promising Spiritual dimension of higher experience. The practice leads towards ultimate reality i.e. Brahman.

In Jnana yoga in the experience of Antaranga the first one is Sravana which means hearing. The practitioner has to go first through an extensive and intensive study, for which one should go to his guru (the spiritual teacher of master) and should listen to the lesson on (about) Brahman.

In ancient time it was done in ashrams (the traditional school of Vedanta or yoga, now-a-days it includes thorough studies of the traditional doctrines of the Vedantic texts or Upanisads. This gives to the mind of the aspirant the right direction and outlook and material for the second stages which is Manana. Manana stars with intellectual analysis of the material gained by studying the texts. The analysis of the material gained by knowledge of the world of sensual and emotional experience and on the level of speculative thinking, final knowledge cannot be found. Absolute truth can lie only beyond them. When the practitioner firmly arrives at this conclusion, he is able to enter the path of meditation which brings him to the following and final stage of training which is Nishisyasana.

This expression can be translated as constant meditation. This stage of training makes it clear to the Sadhaka that the process of opening a new channel to reality over and above the senses and the intellect is not a matter or mental exercises during meditational session only, but it is also an equally necessary to introduce a kind of meditation attitude towards one's life so that eventfully the mind is in a state of meditation even when dealing with the business of everyday life.

Significance of Jnana Yoga

- Discrimination between the real and the unreal
- Renunciation
- Longing for freedom
- Control of the body and the senses
- Control of the mind
- Prevention of the sense-organs, once they are controlled, from drifting back to their respective objects
- Forbearance
- Complete concentration & faith
- Self-control
- Longing for freedom[16]

Through the practice of **forbearance**, the Yogis remain unruffled by heat and cold, pleasure and pain, and the other pairs of opposites. By means of concentration, he keeps his mind on the ideal. Faith enables him to listen, with respect to the instruction of the teacher and the injunctions of the scriptures. This faith is not mechanical belief, but an affirmative attitude of mind regarding the existence of reality, as opposed to a negative and cynical attitude. The man who always doubts comes to a grief.[17]

---

[16] Retrieved on 04.10.2014 [http://www.hinduism.co.za/jnana-.htm]
[17] Retrieved on 04.10.2014 [http://yoga108.org/pages/show/55-jnana-yoga-introduction]

CHAPTER - 5

KARMA YOGA

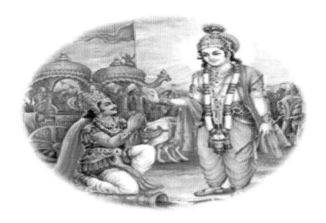

Figure No. 4 Karma Yoga [18]

The Karma comes from Sanskrit root 'Kri' which means to do karma literary means action, which everyone performs in this world, whether consciously or unconsciously. The human beings have a natural tendency to perform some thing. The Gita say:

Na Hi Kascit Ksanamapi Jatu Tistatya Karmart/
Karyate Hyavasab Karma Sarvab Prakrtijairgunaib//

Meaning: No person can stop his activity at any time even for a moment, because the entire humanity has been forced by the nature to perform action. [19]

---

[18] Retrieved on 04.10.2014
[http://www.indianetzone.com/photos_gallery/12/karmayoga-gita_18080.jpg]

Karma is the expression of the rule of perfect justice within us. It is the law of the cosmos reflected in the microcosm. There I nothing arbitrary or punitive about it. It is universal law and inevitable fact. All the phenomena o nature are governed by one important law, the universal law of causation, which is also known by the name ' the law of karma' the law of causation is a universal law that keeps up the inner harmony and the logical order of the universe. Man's deeds are subject to this law.

No success can be attained without understanding the laws of Karma. The three aspects of the law of karma should clearly be grasped. The first is the Sanchita karma, the sum total and stored actions, good or bad in the innumerable past lives that we have left behind. The whole of it is recorder and preserved the second is Prarbdha karma, the inevitable karma. It is that portion of our karma which is assigned to us to be worked out in a single life in relation to men and things we met and experienced in previous lives. The third form is that of Krivamana karma. It is that karma which is in the course of making. It is that which preserves our free-will with certain limitations and ensures our future success.

One cannot do anything with past karmas unless he is folly enlightened. With knowledge of the divine, the enlightened ones cerate the fore of knowledge that burns all the bondages created by past karmas. That is possible but unless one has that ability, he has to reap the consequences of his past karmas.

---

19 K. Kumar; (2009), *Super Science of Yoga,* p.p. 136-140, Standard Publishers (India) New Delhi

Since birth to death the human being karma because of the bondage of the law of karma. These karmas are the causative factor behind the bondage of a person. Now the question arise- if Karma binds us and without doing karma on cannot stop himself then how can one be liberated; or there is no chance? The answer is- as the karmas is the causative factor of bondage, it can liberate the aspirant because it is the causative factor of liberation also. The second question arises what type of karma bounds us and what kind of karma can liberate? Lord Krishna reply's Arjuna in the Gita as:

Tasmachchhastram Pramanam Te Karvakaryavy-Avasthtau/
Jnatwa Sastravidhanoktam Karma Kartumiharhasi//

- **Srimadhbhagvad gita 16/24**

Meaning: Which karma should be performed and which one should not, to distinguish it there is no reference in any text and you should act after knowing the view of authorized text.

One should perform karma according to the need of the situation; the main thing is that one should be aware of his Kartavya (duty). One should perform his duty without any expectation. In this context the Gita says:

Yajnatrthatkarmano'nyatra Loko'yarn Karmaban-Dhanab/
Tadartham Karma Kaunteya Muktasangah Samacharah//

- **Srimadhbhagvad gita 3/9**

Meaning: The world is bound by actions other than those performed for the sake of Yagya, therefor O son of Kunti, you perform action for Yahga only. Her Yagya means the action done for the sake of others or of selfless motive. The Karma performed for others without any expectation, does not bind the aspirant. This selfless action is called karma yoga.

In the first stage of the Sadhana of Karma Yoga the aspirant performs his action with the feeling of duty. Through the attachment to karma or the result of karma the person gets budded with the karma. Hine any obstacle in the path of karma hurts the performer because the performer is attached the fruits of Karma. When the aspirant gives up the attachment to the result he then becomes a karma yogi:

Yuktah Karmaphalam Tyaktya Santimapnoti Majsthikin/
Ayuktab Kamakarna Phale Sakto Nibadhyate//

- **Srimadhbhagvad gita5/12**

Meaning: The aspirant of karma yoga performs the karma for the realization without expectation whereas the Sakam Pursa (general performer) binds them with the desire of result. Hence the karma yogi does not attach himself to the success or failure. Without expectation the mind becomes desire less and then he becomes free from attachments with the world it may lead to liberation.

The question arises now – without expectation can the performer become inspiration less? But the answer in no.

hence the real inspiration will be with the desire less performer. To perform the duty without any obstruction the aspirant needs some code of conducts, which seems to be very difficult but with the help of guru it becomes easier for the karma yogi. In the practice of karma yoga the aspirant needs a guru. In who he has, full faith. It is also important here that the aspirant should have strength of resolution and full dedication to his guru. The faith and resolution makes the path of yoga easier.

Mantra- Chudamanyopnisad says that the disciple should have the following characteristic features with him: the pure mind a good character, faith in guru, dedication to the path and he should be an optimist, with all these virtues the aspirant of karma yoga becomes closer to the god he becomes able to perform the karma and offer it to god, which is the theme of karma yoga. Lord Krishna says the same thing in the Gita as:

Yatkarosi Yadanasi Yajjuhosi Dadasi Yat/
Yatta Pasyasi Kaunteya Tatkurswa Madarpnanm//

- **Srimadhbhagvad gita 9/27**

Meaning: O' son of Kunti (O'Arjun) whatever action you perform like Yagna. Tapa or Dana, offer it to me and then you will be free from the bondage of their results.

Karma yoga in real sense makes one get the freedom which is the goal of human hearing. Every unselfish action takes us towards the goal. Most of the human hens in this world follow. The path of karma yoga consciously or unconsciously. Those who know that the path of karma is like worship of the lord, perform their actions skilfully, selflessly, and lovingly.

It is very effective and valid path of yoga in order to experience the total self. One who is in control of the self and which is devoid of desire is a true enunciate. A true enunciate easily attains enlightenment in this path.

Significance of Karma Yoga

There is extraordinary power in the selfless and desire less *Karma Yoga*. It richly blesses both the individual and the society. A Karma Yogi, who follows his Swadharma, does get his daily bread. Besides, his industriousness makes his body healthy and pure. His work also contributes to the well-being and prosperity of the society in which he lives. Actions done in the pursuit of Swadharma will confer nothing but benefit on the community. A society which has in its midst such Karmoyogis who have identified themselves with those around them, forgetting their selfish interests, will have prosperity, order and harmony.

Work of a Karma Yogi helps sustain him. It keeps his body healthy and intellect radiant. It results in the welfare of the society as well. It also confers on the Karma *Yogi* a great gift in the form of the purity of his mind. It purifies the mind and it is only the clean and pure mind which receives true knowledge. A Karma Yogi's work ultimately leads to the attainment of wisdom. Karma Yogis gained true knowledge through the terms used in their respective vocations. To them, their vocations were like schools of the spirit. Their work was imbued with the spirit of worship and service.

Another great gain that flows from the actions of a Karma Yogi is that a model is place before the society.

As a Karma Yogi finds joy in the work itself, he is ever-absorbed in his work. Hypocrisy does not, therefore, gain ground in the society. A Karma Yogi is happy and content with fulfilment; still he continues to work.[20]

The *Karma Yogi* reaches the summit of spiritual liberation using the ladder of work. He does not kick off that ladder even thereafter. He just cannot do so. Doing work becomes his nature. He thus continues to impress on the society the importance of service in the form of work enjoined by Swadharma.

In short, a *Karma Yogi,* by renouncing desire for the fruit of his actions, will receive infinite rewards. His body will be sustained and both his body and mind will remain healthy and radiant. The society to which he belongs will also be happy and contented. His mind will be purified and he will attain wisdom. The spread of hypocrisy in the society will be precluded, and the sacred ideal will become clear to all. Such is the glory of *Karma Yoga*, which is testified by experience.

Karma Yoga alone is sufficient to lead us to the path of mystical knowledge. Karma Yoga acts as the base for the aspirants of all the other paths of Yoga also.

This is the great strength of Karma Yoga: it promises realization to all. It elevates and ennobles life, and it shows us that there is no need to abandon the world and live in a forest in order to acquire knowledge. Because of Karma Yoga, the other paths of Yoga do not remain an exclusive preserve of ascetics, but are open to all.

Karma Yoga also says that when we work without attachment, we produce the best work. This is the most

---

[20] Retrieved on 04.10.2014
[http://www.mkgandhi.org/talksongita/chap03.htm]

important aspect of Karma Yoga for our practical lives, because it gives us a guide to being the most efficient producer and supplier of work. Normally, when we are thinking of other things, we naturally cannot give full attention to work, and our work cannot be as efficient. But if we can avoid thinking of anything else, if we can avoid thinking even of how and why we are doing the work and how it will benefit us, and concentrate instead on doing whatever we are doing to the best extent possible, then the work that we produce is naturally of a far higher order.

In this principle, Karma Yoga differs from many modern-day coaches, who teach their wards to visualize the final point of success, of crossing the finishing line first and so on. In Karma Yoga, such visualization of the result is not advocated and instead, according to its principles, the trainee should concentrate on the particular training that he or she is receiving at that moment without thinking of the final result. [21]

Karma yoga must not be seen solely as a path connected to religion. Through the ages and in cultures around the world, the methods of karma yoga have been understood and followed by great personalities in their achievements. The need for total absorption in the work itself and the strength that can be derived from it has been understood by scientists, philosophers, artists like musicians, painters, sculptors, etc. from time immemorial. Hence this is not a special secret of yoga but a universal

---

[21] ibid www.mkgandhi.org

truth. It is only that in Hinduism these methods have been employed in spirituality also to attain a mystical end.

Karma yoga is the path for the people of action, the practical people. In the doctrines of the other Yoga, a worldly life is inimical to further knowledge, and it bars those living a worldly life from their spiritual goals. The only way to a spiritual end would be through a complete abandoning of worldly life. But karma yoga shows that the same goals can be attained through a worldly life. It shows us how to tackle the infinite diversions that affect a practical life, and how to fulfil our duties and responsibilities in such a way that work it-self leads us to realization.

The effort is to do perfect work, but not expect anything from it, and hence not gets attached to it. Once the work is finished, we should be able to rise up from it without thinking about it anymore. Work itself becomes a meditation, and through work we attain our liberty.

Karma yoga by itself can lead us to realization, but it also forms the underpinning for those who follow the path of Bhakti, Raja yoga and Gyan yoga, for fulfilling their duties. Even yogis have to do work as long as they are alive, and hence karma yoga is essential for all. This path shows us how to use the world with all its diversions to work out our way to spiritual goals.

Karma yoga says, our duty is whatever is enjoined and we find in our particular position and situation in life. Sometimes a particular act which is appropriate in one situation might turn out to be wrong in another. These are everyday problems faced by all in society because of its conflicting nature, and it is difficult then to know how to act. Karma yoga lays down a general rule to guide us in all such situations, which is to perform that action which is Sattvic and to avoid that which is Rajasic or Tamasic.[22]

Karma yoga instead shows us how to achieve moral guidelines by changing our personality. It tells us, not *what* to do, but *how* to do it. It teaches us to have always a Sattvic attitude, free from cruelty, lust, anger, etc. If we can maintain Sattva, then we will automatically know what action to do in a particular situation.[23]

[22] ibid www.mkgandhi.org
[23] ibid www.mkgandhi.org

CHAPTER - 6

RAJA YOGA

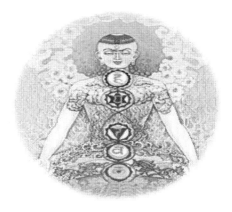

Figure No. 5 Raja Yoga [24]

The word raja yoga is found in many of the Upanishads. It may be regarded as the master of all the yogic practices. All the yogic practices lead to Samadhi, but the specialty of this path is that it starts from, Samadhi. Hence the Samadhi comes in every path, thus it has been considered to be the complimentary practice of yoga or the greatest path of yoga.[25]

The importance of raja yoga has been accepted very widely the great hatha yogi Swatmaram also says in Hatha Prodipika as:

---

[24]   Retrieved   on   04.10.2014   [http://4.bp.blogspot.com/--B1TEfRnH38/TpdXg-KBrD_kAHo/s1600/raja_yoga.jpg]

[25] S.S. Saraswati; (2013), *Four Chapter on Freedom,* p.p.7, Yoga Publications Trust, Munger, Bihar, India

41

Kevalam rajyogaya hathavidyopnidisyate//

-Hatha Pradipika

Meaning: The lesion of hatha yoga is only for the attainment of raja yoga.

There are various definitions of Raja Yoga, Yoga Swarodaya defines it as:

**Yathakase Bharaman Vayurakas Vrajate Svayam/
Tathakase Manolina Rajayoga Krivamatam//**

Meaning: Just as air passing through sky never appears likewise to establish the mind in Sunya (no object) is raja yoga.

Yogasikhopanisad defines raja yoga as:

Rajso Retso yogadrajyoga iti smritah//

Meaning: The *Raj* form of Kundalini when merges with *Ret* form of give or the union of *Atma tattwa* (individual self) with *Brahma Tattwa* (the supreme self) is Raja Yoga.

A careful observation of the above mentioned definitions shows that the establishment of the self in Brahman is Raja Yoga. In this state the practitioner becomes one with Brahman; the dualism destroys and this is the aim of any path of Yoga. For the practitioner the world disappears; and the; practitioner gets rid of all miseries of the world and he IS established in the self.

The practitioner of Raja Yoga has been divided into three kinds: the first type is *Uttam* or the advance practitioner,

42

second type of Raja Yogi is called *Madhyam* or the medium and the third one is called *Adham* or the beginners. This categorisation also differentiates the practice of the individual.[26]

The *Urtam* type of practitioner needs a special type of. package for the Attainment that is *Abhyas* and *Vairagya.* Mahargi Patanjali has also given the same instruction to them in his Yoga Sutra :

Abhyas Vairagyabhyam Tannirodhah //

- Patanjali 'Yoga Sutra 1/12

Meaning: There are two methods for stopping the flow of the Chitta Virttis. First is Abhyasa or continuous practice and the second one is Vairagya or detachment from all the rage and Dwesa (liking and disliking).

The next thing is Iswarpranidhan, it has been said that the advance practitioner can attain the Samadhi through *Iswarpranidhan* only. In this context Maharsi Patanjali says in his Yoga Sutra:

Samadhi Siddhiriswar Pranidhanat//

- **Patanjali yoga sutra 2/45**

Meaning: One can attain success in Samadhi by complete resignation/surrender to god. Here they would Samadhi is not exactly that; it is a state of trance. In this

---

26 K. Kumar; (2009), *Super Science of Yoga,* p.p. 141-145, Standard Publishers (India) New Delhi

state the aspirant loses the body awareness and becomes able to start with deeper awareness.

Hence the aspirant is here of high quality, they need not to practice the other steps; they can starts from Samadhi onward. Such yogis already have completed their sadhana in past lives.

The second type of practitioner (Madhyam) has been instructed to practice Kriya Yoga. This type of aspirant needs a few more hard practices as they also have past life practice but in lower form. Thus for them Patanjali describes Kriya Yoga as:

Tapah Swadhyayaeswarpranidhani Kryayogan//

- **Patanjali yoga sutra 2/1**

Meaning: Tapa (penance) Swadhyay (self-study) and Iswarpranidhan (faith in fod) constitutes Kriya Yoga. Tapa literary means to burn, here Tapah means the Sadhana of optimum level where all the past karma burns and the aspirant illuminates the imperfection.

The aspirant of medium class needs to develop the mastery over summer-winter, pain-pleasure. And contempt-respect etc. the mind then becomes able to be stable in all the stages. Aspirant starts studying the self the inner self (Swadhyaya) and it leads towards surrender to god (Iswarpranidhan) these three things lead the aspirant to attain the Samadhi.

The beginners or ham Sadhaka those who did not start the Sadhana has been suggested to adopt Astanga yoga (eight fold path). Manarsi Patanjali says in his yoga sutra:

Yamaniyamasanapranayamaprayyaharadharan a Dhyansmadhayostavangani//

- **Patanjali yoga sutra 2/29**

Meaning: Yama, Niyama, Asana, Pranayama, Pratyahara, Dharana, Dhyan and Samadhi are the steps of Astanga Yoga they need to practice all the steps as their body and mind both need a preparation and suppleness for Samadhi.

In the practice of raja yoga the aspirant requires the practice to attain the Samadhi according to his level. Somewhere raja yoga is also known as Dhyan Yoga because ultimately the aspirant has to reach that state where Samadhi is easier to attain. In this context Dharana, Dhyan and Samadhi come in series and are called Samayama together:

Trayamkaetra samyamah //

- *Patanjali Yoga Sutra ¾*

Meaning: When Dharana (concentration), Dhyan (meditation) and Samadhi becomes one this state is called Samyama or discipline is, necessary, no doubt but at the same time regularity too, it essential for the aspirant.

Now the question arises if the every Sadhaka or aspirant has to reach Samadhi only then what is the difference among them? There are different levels of

Samadhi too, which has been suggested to different levels of Sadhaka (aspirant).

We have the description of the four kinds of raja yogi in ancient texts. They are as follows: the first is asthma kalmia, the second one is Madhu Bhumika and the third and is Madhu Pratika and the fourth is Atikaran Bhanaiya among them Pratham Kalpita is said to be the newly arrived they need to practice the Savitarka Samadhi. The second type of yogi which is said to be at better level the Madhu Bhumika, they need to have the practice of Nirvitarka Samadhi. The third type of raja yogi which is known as Madhu Bhumika and said to be better than both of them need to practice the Asmitanugata Samadhi. The best level of Sadhaka or Atikrant Bhananiya Yogi has already attained the mastery over Ritambhara-Prajna and over Asmitanutata Samadhi. Through the regular practice of that he experiences Asampragyat Samadhi.

When the Sadhaka or aspirant becomes able to govern the Gitavriti (mental fluctuation) of mind and attain Ritambhara.-Prajna. He becomes one with his Karana Prakriti or the subtle self and atman gets liberated and thus attains the Kaivalya the ultimate reality).

Thus it can be said that raja yoga is the only practice of yoga which is open for all and easier to adopt also only through the practice of raja yoga. Atman becomes able to know the real self.

Significance of Raja Yoga

Raja means King. A king acts with independence, self-confidence and assurance. Likewise, a Raja Yogi is autonomous, independent and fearless. Raja Yoga is the path of self-discipline and practice.

Raja Yoga is also known as Ashtanga Yoga (Eight Steps of Yoga), because it is organized in eight parts:

i. Yama - Self-control
ii. Niyama - Discipline
iii. Asana - Physical exercises
iv. Pranayama - Breath exercises
v. Pratyahara - Withdrawal of the senses from external objects
vi. Dharana - Concentration
vii. Dhyana - Meditation
viii. Samadhi - Complete Realization

The eight steps of Raja Yoga provide systematic instruction to attain inner peace, clarity, self-control and Realization.[27]

Other benefits of Raja Yoga: [28]

- Gain freedom from stress and anxiety.
- Create a sense of well-being.
- Enhance memory and concentration.
- Mind becomes more clear and focused.
- Overcome negative habits.
- Improve quality of sleep.

---

[27] Retrieved on 04.10.2014 [http://www.yogaindailylife.org]
[28] Retrieved on 04.10.2014 [http://www.brahmakumaris.org]

CHAPTER - 7

HATHA YOGA

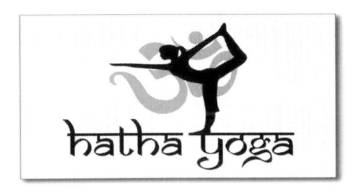

Figure No. 6 Hatha Yoga [29]

Normally people understand hatha yoga means the practice of yogic postures forcefully, whether it takes lot of energy or makes the practitioner exerted. But it is definitely not the same. The word 'hatha' has been used in yogic texts and ancient literature in a different meaning. It has been defined as:

Kakara Kirtitah Suryasya Thakara Chandra Uchyate/ Surya Chandra Measauryogad Hathayogo Nimadyate//

Meaning: The word 'hatha' is made up of two Bija mantras: 'Ha' and 'Tha' where 'Ha' represents Sun or Pingala Nadi and 'Tha' represents Moon or Ida Nadi. Basically the union of these two Nadies is called hatha

---

[29] Retrieved on 04.10.2014
[http://rlv.zcache.com/lord_of_the_dance_pose_hatha_yoga_post_cards
-r015cff0daafb423fa000f6f82e3f20b2_vgbaq_8byvr_512.jpg]

yoga. The meaning of these two Bija can be understood as follows; 'Tha' represents Prana, the vital energy and 'ha' represents mental energy. So hatha yoga means the union to the Pranic and mental forces.[30]

When Ida and Pingala unites together the Prana starts following into Susumna and the dormant power Kundalini which is lying in the Muladhara chakra, rises and enters Susumna and passing through all the six chakras reaches the highest peak Brahmarandhra or Sahauraua and attain the oneness. This is the union of Sakti and Siva or Atman and Parmatman, this process destroys the ignorance of the aspirant and illuminates his heart and soul. Thus the process of this union is called yoga.

The aim of hatha yoga is to have the mastery over body and mind. The main objective is to create an absolute balance of the interacting activities and processes of the physical body, mind and energy. When this balance is established the impulses generated give a call of awakening to the central force which is responsible for the evolution of human consciousness.

There are various texts of hatha yoga. Among them Hatha Pradipika by Swatmarama and Gheranda Samhita by Maharsi Gheranda are more important. According to Swatmanma the evolution process of Hatha Yoga includes Asama, Pramayama. Mudra-Bandha and Nadanusandhan whereas Gheranda Samhita another test of hath yoga explains the process in seven in details as:

---

[30] K. Kumar; (2009), *Super Science of Yoga*, p.p. 146-151, Standard Publishers (India) New Delhi

Sidahnam Dridhatachaiva Sthairya Dharryam Ch Laghavm /
Pratyaksam Ca Nirliptam Ghatastha Sapta Sadhanam//

Meaning: These are the following steps: Sodhanam (purification), Dridhta (suppleness of body), Sthairya (stillness of body), Dhairyam (patience), Laghavam (lightness of body) Pratyaksam (facing the troubles) and Nirliptam (detachment) of Ghatastha Sapta Sadhan (seven steps of the perfection of body) which should be practiced by the aspirant o hatha yoga.

How to attain this perfection, for that Maharsi Gheranda explains the Saptanga Yoga (7 steps of yoga) as:

Satkarmna Sodhanam Ca Asanena Bhaved Dredham/
Mudraya Sthirta Caiva Pratyaharena Dhirata//

Pranayam Laghavam Ca Dhyanat Pratyaksam Atmane/
Samadhinam Ca Nirliptam Mukti Raiva Na Sansayh//

Meaning: The practice of Satkarma purifies the body. Asana makes the body strong, mudras bring stillness in the body; through the practice of Pratyahara one can get the patience. Pranayame makes the body of Sadhaka of aspirant light and by the practice of Samadhi the mind gets detached; there is no doubt about it.

The above mentioned seven steps of yoga should be understood in detail. Hatha yoga is also known as the science of purification as it includes six types of cleansing process. In order to purity the mind it is necessary for the body as a whole to undergo a process of absolute purification. This purification or Satkarma are: Dhauti,

Neti, Basti, Nauli, Trataka, and Kapalbhati. Here is the brief introduction of all six processes of purification.

Maharsi Gherand explains the Satkarma very systematically. The first Satkarma is Dhauti. This means to lean and in Gheranda Samhita it is said to be of four types: Antaradhauti, Dantadhauti, Hridadhauti and Mulasodhan.

Antardhauti literally means internal organs cleansing. It is of four types again. Which are Vatsar, Varisar, Vahnisar and Bahiskrita. Danta Dhauti means dental cleansing which is also of four types: Danta mula, Jihwa mula, Karnarandhra and Kapalrandhra, Hrida Dhauti means cleansing of heart region and it is of three types: Danda Dhauti Vaman Dhauti and Vastra Dhauti. The fourth Dhauti is Mula Sodhana, which is the cleansing of anal region.

The second process is Neti. It should be understood as the nasal passage cleansing. Basically it is of two types: Jala Neti and Sutra Neti according to Ghreranda Samhita. Somewhere there is the description of Dugdha Neti and Ghrita Neti.

The next cleansing process is Basti. It is the cleansing of lower abdomen or rectum only. It is of two types according to Maharsi Gheranda: Jala Basti and Pawan Basti.

Later the practice comes is Nauli. It is the movement of abdominal muscles and it is of three types: Daksina nauti, Vama Nauli and Madhya Nauli.

Trataka is the cleaning of eyes. According to Gheranda Samhita it is of two types: Vahya ans Abhyantar.

The last process is Kaplabhati and it is also of three types: Vatakrama, Sitakarma and Vyutakarma.

Practice of Satkarma mentioned above is not necessary for all aspirants: it is for those who need the inner cleansing. This means the aspirant doesn't have balanced three Dosa (Vata, Pitta and Kapha) or Sapta Dhatus are not in balance. The practice of Satkarma brings a balance among them.

After the practice of Satkarma the practice comes in Hatha Yoga is Asana. Hence Patajjali Yoga Sutra defines Asana as Sthiram Sukham Asanam (stillness and comfortable posture is called Asana) but in hatha yoga it is a specific position which opens the energy channels and psychic centres. When Prana or energy flows freely, the body also becomes supple. Stiffness of the body is due to blockages and accumulation of wastes.

It is said that it should be of eighty-four lacks types but it doesn't seem practical. We find the description of eighty-four-types of Asanas. Maharsi Gheranda describes thirty-two types of Asana. Among them Padmasana, Siddhasana, Swastikasana, Vajrasana, Paschimottansana are common. Siddhasana is said to be the best for Sadhana, as Siddhasana blocks the down fall of energy, it is useful for spiritual awakening.

There after the practice comes in hatha yoga is mudra. Mudra is the specific gesture of the body. Hatha Yoga

Pradipika discusses ten mudras whereas Gherand Samhita mentions twenty-five types of mudra. Jalandhar Bandha, Mula Bandha, Uddiyana bandah, Maha Bandha, Maha mudra, Khechari and Viparitakani Mudra are common among them.

Hatha yogic texts give a lot of importance to the practice of Pranayama. It is very clearly said that for the perfection in Sadhana of Hatha Yoga Pranayama should be practiced after Asanas. Texts describe Astakumbhaka (eight fold practice of Pranayam) i.e. Surya Bhedi, Ujjai, Bhastrika, Bharamari, Sitali, Sitkari, Murchha and Plavini. Through the practice of Pranayama body becomes light weighted, all the Nadies become purified and the mind becomes stable.

Now comes the practice of Dharan, Dhyan and Samadhi; which is the asset of any Sadhana. Practice of Dhyan or meditation is of four types as mentioned in hatha yoga; which are: Padastha, Pindastha, Rupastha and Rupatita. There is the description of two types of specific Meditation. They are Sangma and Nigama Dhyan. Practice of Dhyan leads to self-realization and through the regular practice of that Dhyan the mind becomes detached and it is the state of Samadhi the aspirant can attain the Moksa or Kaivalya. Swami Swatmaram explains the aim of Hatha Yoga in Hatha Pradipika as:

Kivalam Rajyogaya Hthavidyopnidisyate//

- **Hatha Pradipika**

Meaning: The lesson of hatha yoga is only for the attainment of raja yoga or the ultimate reality.

The same thing is repeated at the end of the text as follows:

Sarve Hathyopaya Rajayogasya Siddhayae//

-   **Hatha Pradipika 4/103**

Meaning: All the practices and clues given in hatha yoga is only for the attainment of raja yoga.

Significance of Hatha Yoga

Hatha Yoga for All Ages

Whatever age you might be or whatever your state of mind, you are sure to find yoga fun and beneficial. You might be young or old, fit or ailing, there will be an asana out there that will be suitable for you and will successfully make you fitter and stronger.

Children and teenagers find it relatively easy to pick up the Asana of hath yoga as they have a body that is extremely flexible. Along with retaining and improving their flexibility, children can improve their co-ordination and concentration and it can also help them develop a sense of discipline.

Pregnant women also find yoga an ideal form of exercise. Being relatively gentle, with fluid and non-jerky movements, yoga reduces backache that is common in this condition. Women who regularly practiced yoga found their labor pains to be shorter and less intensive.

For older people, yoga brings flexibility, better posture, a stronger spine, and better blood circulation, subsequently getting rid of back pain, indigestion, and breathing disorders.

The Physical Benefits of Hatha Yoga

The physical benefits of hatha yoga have been acknowledged by many people all over the world. Practicing the various postures, stretching your body and regulating your breathing brings with it several benefits for your body. It's a well-known fact that it improves the overall flexibility of the body. Apart from this, it improves your balance, corrects your posture and gives you strong and well-toned muscles. Circulation of blood increases in the body relieving you of muscle pain and making you feel fresh and energized.[31]

There are a lot of people who take to hatha yoga to lose weight and get a better body. Even though yoga doesn't increase the heart rate for a long duration of time, it can tone and tighten the muscles, thereby improving your looks.

Mental Benefits of Hatha Yoga

Hatha yoga goes a long way in relaxing the mind, and makes it strong enough to fight stress. You are able to concentrate and focus better and you'll find yourself becoming a calmer and less agitated person. It increases one's awareness about the body and clears the mind of all kinds of negativity. If there are any chronic stress patterns in your body, hatha yoga helps to relieve them.

Hatha yoga empowers you to cope with all the hassles of a modern day life. The deep breathing exercises taught in hatha yoga can be done anytime and anywhere and they recharge your body and mind almost instantaneously.[32]

---

[31] Retrieved on 04.10.2014
[http://www.hathayogaillustrated.com/benefits-of-hatha-yoga/]
[32] ibid www.hathayogaillustrated.com

Benefits of a regular Hatha Yoga practice

- Makes the body stronger and more flexible.
- Release tension and trauma stored in the body.
- Calms the mind.
- Creates space in body and mind and in that space you find 'balance' and the opportunity for spiritual growth.[33]

---

[33] Retrieved on 04.10.2014 [http://www.ekhartyoga.com/everything-yoga/yoga-styles/hatha-yoga]

CHAPTER - 8

DHYANA YOGA

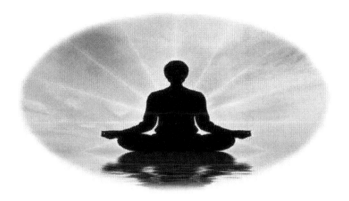

Figure No. 7 Dhyana Yoga [34]

What is real meaning of Dhyana (meditation)? It is a state of pure consciousness, which transcends the inner and outer senses. The word meditation is derived from two Latin words: meditari (to think, to dwell upon and to exercise the mind) and meditari (to heal). Meditation usually refers to a state in which the body is consciously relaxed and the mind is allowed to become calm and focused.

The climax of Dhyana is Samadhi, in Indian tradition, it is used for inner soul illumination, and western psychologists link it with a special state of mind. The

---

[34] Retrieved on 04.10.2014
[http://cdn6.bigcommerce.com/sjr4nh8s/product_images/uploaded_images/samadhi.jpg?t=140732028]

techniques and nature of meditation may vary but modern scientific researches validate and highlight its benefits. The practice of meditation helps in building up the coping ability. The practitioner of meditation slowly becomes aware of the inherent dormant potentialities and thus prevents himself from becoming a victim of distress.[35]

Mahrsi Patanjali had disclosed the secret of controlling the mind in his yoga-sutra five thousand years ago as; **"Yogaschittavrittinirodhah"** yoga is retraining the mind stuff (chitta) from taking various forms (vrittis). Practice of meditation is one of the important steps of eight fold path of yoga, guided by Patanjali:

Des Bandhasya Cittasya Dharana //
- **Patanjali Yoga Sutra 3/1**

The mind tries to think of one object, to hold itself to one particular point, e.g. The top of the head, the heart, etc., and if the mind succeeds in receiving the sensations only through that part of the body, that would be dharma (concentration), and when mind succeeds in keeping itself in that state for some time, it is called Dhyana (meditation). Maharsi Patanjali defines Dhyan as:

Tatra Prtyaiktanta Dhyanam//
- **Patanjali yoga sutra 3/2**

Meaning: Uninterrupted stream of the content of consciousness is Dhyan (meditation). In other words

---

35 K. Kumar; (2009), *Super Science of Yoga,* p.p. 152-159, Standard Publishers (India) New Delhi

practice of Dharana of concentration when becomes prolonged and uninterrupted it becomes meditation.

Dhyan according to the Gita is a practice of self-purification through which the aspirant controls the functioning of senses and mind. Lord Krishna describes the process and the importance of the meditation in the sixth chapter of Gita as:

Samarth Kayasirogrivam Dharayannaclam Sthirah/
Sampreksya Nasikagram Svam Desascanavalokayan//

- Srimadh Bhagwd Gita 6/13

Prasantatma Vigaabhibrabmacarivrate Sthitab/
Manah Sam,Yama Maccito Yucta Asita Matparah//

- Srimadh Bhagwd Gita 6/14

Yunjannegvam Sadatmanam Yogi Nivatamansab/
Santim Nirvanparman Mastsamsthamadhigacchati//

- Srimadh Bhagwd Gita 6/15

Meaning: Keep the head neck and spine straight and steady and bring the awareness on the tip of the nose. Don't lose the concentration during the practice. Firm in the vow of complete chastity and fearless, keep oneself perfectly calm and with the mind held in restraint, fixed on me (god). Constantly apply the mind to me (god), the aspirant of such disciplined mind attains everlasting peace, consisting of supreme bliss, which abides in me (the supreme consciousness).

Dhyan according to Swami Vivekananda is a state of mind when it has been trained to remain fixed on a certain internal or external location, there comer to it the power of flowing in an unbroken current, as it were towards that point. He writes in his book Raja Yoga-that if the mind can first concentrate upon an object and is able to continue in that concentration, everything comes under the control of such mind.

Dhyan or meditation according to Swami Sivananda is – to keeping up of flow of one idea like the flow of oil. He writes in Dhyan Yoga that here are two types of meditation which are: concrete and abstract the concrete is for beginners and the abstract is for advance practitioner.

Pandit Sriram Sharma Acharya (1976) in a Sadhana Camp unfolded the practical aspect of meditation in his words mental concentration on some gross objects e.g. an idol or a picture of a deity, is most convenient for majority of people: because, the human mind, in general, is not so developed that it can be concentrated without any visible or perceptible symbol. However with sincere practice, one begins to realize the presence of spirit in his inner self and learn to meditate upon it.

Even in Vedic Literature, Upanisads, Gita and Puranas, we have the description of meditation. Lord Krishna says to Arjuna in thirty fifth verse of the sixth chapter in The Gita:

Asamsayam Mahabhaho Mano Durnigraham Chalam /
Abhyasen Tu Kaunteya Vairagyen Ca Grhyate //

- *Srimadbhagwad Gita 6/35*

Meaning: The mind is restless no doubt and difficult to curb O'Arjuna; but it can be brought under control by repeated practice of meditation and by the exercise of dispassion O' son of Kunti.

Swami Satyananda states in his text 'Meditation from Tantra' that the meditation is our secret property, which can be realized easily, but the only obstacle is our modern life style. This life style brings us in the state of stress and anxiety. It is only due to ignorance of our own nature. If someone becomes able to make a harmony between them the meditation becomes easy to him.

K. N. Udupta the author of Stress and its management by Yoga suggests that stress-related disorders evolve gradually through four stages. In the first stage, psychological symptoms like anxiety and irritability arise due to over activation of the sympathetic nervous system. Research has shown that hormones and other biochemical compounds in the blood indicative of stress tend to decrease during Meditation practice. These changes also stabilize over time, so that a person is actually less stressed biochemically during daily activity.

Judith Horstman states that meditation can help relieve many arthritis symptoms, such as pain, anxiety, stress and depression. As well as ease the fatigue and insomnia associated with fibromyalgia. It affects many body processes connected with wellbeing and relaxation. Recent studies suggest meditation may balance the immune system to help the body resist disease, and even heal. A study of 28 women with fibromyalgia in 1998 at the University of Maryland found that an eight-week program of mindfulness meditation combined with the Chinese movement therapy *qi gong* and counselling in pain management techniques resulted in significant improvement in pain threshold, depression, coping and function.

Dr. Benson says that the practice of meditation changes the way our brain works, and he has found in his research study that thoughts can influence the brain and the body. When his research team used MRI imaging to study the brains of four people meditating, he says the team found increased activity in specific areas involved in attention and control of the autonomic nervous system.

Andrew Newberg, Psychiatry Resource, University of Pennsylvania has demonstrated a change in brain activity during meditation. Newberg infused a radioactive dye into the blood of eight experienced Tibetan Buddhist meditators to track the blood flow in the brain and light up the most active regions. Meditation allowed their brains to block information from the section of the brain that orients the body in space and time. Their bodies stopped responding to external stimuli and focused their energy inward. Newberg's experiment firmly established that practice of meditation alters brain activity.

Psychosomatic Medicine, in another study demonstrated positive effects on the immune system in participants achieving the shift in brain activity. Researchers at the University of Wisconsin gave flu shots to a group of newly-taught meditators and a control group of non-meditators then measured the antibody levels in their blood. They also tracked brain activity to see how much the meditator's mental activity shifted from the right hemisphere to the left. The meditators blood contained more antibodies after flu shots. The participants whose brain activity shifted the most had even more antibodies.

The results suggest that people who take the time to cultivate their meditation technique will benefit from a healthier immune system. Meditation can also improve irritable bowel syndrome, ulcers, and insomnia, among other stress-related conditions. Eighty percent of the people who use meditation to relieve insomnia are successful. Meditation can help prevent or treat stress-related complaints such as anxiety, headaches and bone, muscle and joint problems. Meditation also provides an inner sense of clarity and calm, and that, in it, may help ward off certain illnesses.

What is the region behind these changes? Meditation regulates and controls electrical and chemical activities in the brain, heart rhythm, blood pressure, skins capacity of resistance and many such functions inside the body. Meditation in real sense is an active hypo metabolic condition.

Psychologists say that in a state of calm and quiet mind a great subtle energy field emerges from the deep recesses of the soul. It is very difficult for the ordinary people to have a feeling of this energy field. A disciplined mind helps in physical, mental and spiritual wellbeing. There an; several techniques of meditation among them *Savita, /Dhyan* (Meditation on rising Sun) is highly effective and beneficial.

How to practice it? Select a well-ventilated calm and clean place for the practice. It will be more effective if the timing is of sunrise. Sit in *Padmasana, Siddhasana* or *Sukhasana* (simple cross legged) with the spine erect and body parts relaxed. After the body part awareness observe the natural flow of breath. Slowly bring the awareness at centre of brain and try to visualize the light spot of rising Sun. After a few days practice the infusion of light in the brain in the mind should inspire the practitioner to become a witness of all the internal experiences.

The first sign of this progress is that — there should be nothing negative or illusive in the mind. All the thoughts should be positive and constructive. In general the human mind is flooded by strong currents of pell-mell thoughts and imaginations, the bedlam of passions and impulses keeps hovering around a drain. Sometimes the mind is boiling in anger: sometimes erotic thoughts perturb it, some moments the mind think of a movie, soon may begin to plan for the purchase of a lottery-ticket and dream about that.

This way the practitioners keep recklessly wasting the mental energy in uselessly purposeless and haphazard imaginations and thoughts. In the words of Pandit Sriram Sharma Acharya: "If you were altering and had focused you mind on analytical thinking and given a focused direction to your thoughts, you would have delved deeper in your selected field of knowledge: some of you would have become a Voltaire by now."

He further states "If you had dived deeper in your psyche and given creative, enlightened direction to your imaginations, you might have been another Ravindranath Tagore. People regard me as an eminent thinker. If it is true, it is only because of one thing: 1 have always focused my thinking faculty in specific directions, towards search for true knowledge. I have controlled my thoughts and imaginations: they never fly randomly. Deep and focused mental concentration is a major prerequisite for meditation."

With regular practice of a balanced series v tech energy of the body and mind can be liberate and of consciousness can be expanded. This is not a subjective claim but is now being investigated by the scientists shown by an empirical fact. Experience of the calming meditation only for 10 minutes each day, would create of physical relief that enhances immune function.

The happiness and peace in human life depend on a living and unshakable faith in our immortal origin in the Divine various methods of meditation, prayer and worship have been designed to nourish and augment this aspiration for manifesting divine life in ourselves.

Significance of Dhyana Yoga

Daily meditation practice brings peace of mind, inner joy and inner peace. By increasingly gaining control over your mind, every session brings you closer and closer to your own Self, the centre of your being filled with joy, wisdom and bliss.

Meditation helps you understand how your mind works, and when you understand how your mind works you can begin to make purposeful changes to your life to improve it. Additionally, meditation improves your ability to objectively analyse your emotions, mental states, thought patterns, and responses to events that occur around you.

"Regular meditation opens the avenues of intuitive knowledge, makes the mind calm and steady, awakens an ecstatic feeling and brings the Yogic students in contact with the source of the Supreme Purusha (God). If there are doubts, they are all cleared by themselves when you march on the path of Dhyana Yoga steadily".

Swami Sivananda

When you meditate regularly your mind becomes clearer and more focused, thereby improving your quality of life and allowing you to perform better and more quickly all tasks you choose to be involved in. Not only can meditation help you reach your goals quicker, but also and more importantly, it can guide you in setting better and wiser goals in life.

There are also numerous benefits for the physical body. Studies have shown that the regular practice of meditation can assist one in lowering blood pressure, decreasing stress, improving memory, and bring in a host of other health benefits.

"You will get the full Ananda (Bliss) of the divine glory only when you merge deep into silent meditation".[36]

Swami Sivananda

John White has enumerated some special benefits of Dhyan as:

1. A feeling of tranquillity and freedom in daily life,
2. Reduction in psychological disorders like anxiety, tiredness and depression etc.,
3. Relief from various pains, such as headache, joint pains etc.,
4. Very beneficial in insomnia;
5. Infinite patience, and increase in affection and sympathy for others;
6. Growth in devotion and belief in the Supreme Being;
7. A stronger urges and aptitude for service and cooperation in social life.[37]

---

[36] Retrieved on 04.10.2014 [http://yoga108.org/pages/show/108-meditation-definition-and-benefits]

[37] Retrieved on 04.10.2014 [http://www.akhandjyoti.org/?Akhand-Jyoti/2004/Sept-Oct/DhyanBenefits/]

CHAPTER - 9

MANTRA YOGA

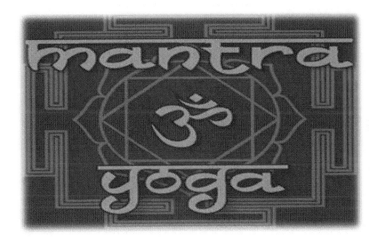

Figure No. 8 Mantra Yoga [38]

Meaning of Mantra: The root *'Man'* in the word Mantra comes from the first syllable of that word, meaning 'to think', and *'Tra'* from *'Trai'* meaning to protect' or 'free' from the bondage of *Samsara* or the phenomenal world. By the combination of *'Man'* and *'Tra'* comes Mantra.

Importance of Mantra: Mantras have great significance in the mental and spiritual evolution of harmony. These could also manifest tremendous results in the physical world; they could be powerful like a Patton tank or an atomic bomb. Our spiritually empowered, Eminent ancestors — *The Rsis,* knew this fact and had

---

[38]Retrieved on 04.10.2014 [http://www.mantrayoga.com.au/wp-content/themes/mantra-blue-theme/images/header_image.jpg]

therefore developed a whole gamut of mantras for specific purposes and had also devised the methods experimentation with the use of these subliminal tools.[39]

History of Mantra: Mantras also have their own history of discovery and mastery of inner realms of consciousness by a long line of masters and seekers of spirit. Mantras and Yantras have been in existence since prehistoric times. The Vedic scriptures describe that once the Devas (gods) and the Asuras (demons) argued as to what was superior - *mantra* or *Yantra*? The demons regarded Yantras as superior and mightier as material resources and capabilities were more important to them. The gods affirmed the prominence of mantras; that is, spirituality was of greater significance to them. We all have seen and used several types of Yantras in this age of materialistic progress. Let us acquaint ourselves with some knowledge of mantras here.

Effect of Mantras: The effects of mantras largely pertain to the mental, emotional and spiritual realms of life. Mantras inspire positive and penetrating thoughts and enlighten the emotional and deeper levels of consciousness. **'Mananat-trayate iti Mantrah'** - By the Manana (constant thinking or recollection) of which one is protected or is released from the round of births and deaths, is Mantra. That is called Mantra by the meditation (Manana) on which the Jiva or the individual soul attains freedom from sin, enjoyment in heaven and final liberation, and by the aid of which it attains in full the fourfold fruit *(Chaturvarga)*. i.e., *Dharma,*

---

[39] K. Kumar; (2009), *Super Science of Yoga,* p.p. 160-169, Standard Publishers (India) New Delhi

Artha. Kama and *Moksa.* A Mantra is so called because it is achieved by the mental process.

Mantras are very special configurations of sounds or syllables. Accordingly, each mantra has specific patterns of enunciation or chanting. Mantras work on the Yantra of our physical body and also on our energy-body, mind and the inner-self. In the Mantra Yoga meditation one has to chant a word or a phrase until he/she transcends mind and emotions. In the process the super conscious is discovered and achieved. The rhythm and the meaning of mantras combine to conduct the mind safely back to the point of meditation- the higher consciousness or-the specific spiritual focus. Different syllables, phrases and words possess their unique healing potential. Hence they are chanted at a specific time. As a tool to achieve stillness, the mantra is to be discarded at the moment stillness is achieved. Sometimes mantras are also applied to modify circumstances. In the chanting of the mantras it is of immense importance that they are pronounced properly or else all their intended effect would not come. For such purposes it is important that the proper pronunciation is imparted.

The phonemes of the Vedic hymns and the seven fundamental nodes —Sa, Re, Ga, Ma, Pa, Dha, Ni of the Indian classical music have originated (distinctly recognized by the Rrsis) from the vibrations of the sublime sound of Om in the Nature. The Vedic quote— **'Ekoham Bahusyami'** implies that all the sounds, all the energies, all the motions and everything existing in the universe .have originated from the vibrations of this single anahata nada.

This is the source of the manifestation of the *Sabda-Brahm* and the *Nada Brahm*.

Uses of Mantras: Mantras are in the form of praise and appeal to the deities, craving for help and mercy. Some Mantras control and command the evil spirits. Rhythmical vibrations of sound give rise to forms. Recitation of the Mantras gives rise to the formation of the particular figure of the deity.

There are several ways to practice Mantra Yoga. Repeat the Mantra verbally for some time, in a whisper for some time and mentally for some time. The mind wants variety. It gets disgusted with any monotonous practice. The mental repetition is very powerful. It is termed *Manasika Japa*. The verbal or loud repetition is called *Vaikhari Japa*. The loud Japa shuts out all worldly sounds. There is no break of Japa here Repetition in a whisper or humming is termed *Upansu Japa*. Even mechanical repetition of Japa without any Bhava has a great purifying effect on the heart or the mind. The feeling will come later on when the process of mental purification goes on.

Mantras are not some verbal structures to be enunciated rhythmically and repeatedly. Rather, these are subtle means of contemplating that can reorient the mental tendencies &. Many people suffer from a variety of adversities, scarcities and worries because they do not have the aptitude to be initiated into proper mantras (of sane thinking, righteous attitude etc.). Mantras are defined as the tools for liberation from ignorance, illusion, infirmities and sorrows. These can transform the course of life and convert agonies into joys. Indeed, mantras, as special carriers of the energy of cosmic 'Lund, o haste amazing potentials for affecting the physical world also (as it has been commonly seen or read about mantra based healing of physical and mental ailments. etc.). But the spiritual powers and benefits of the mantras are far more intense creative.

Healing by mantras is an important aspect of the science of occultism. It can provide healing even in incurable diseases remedy personality disorders and enable overcome the greatest of difficulties. The impossible become possible; the unachievable is made achievable. The true adepts in the theory and practice of this science are able the powers of nature favourably and positively modifying the course of destiny.

Types of Mantras: Many define mantra as an uplifting, energy- charged sublimated thought current. For example, Gayatri Mantra is the most sacred and sublime thought in the whole creation in it. Prayer has been made to the divine symbolized as sun on behalf of whole of humanity for the gifts of righteousness and enlightened intelligence. "**Om Burbhuvah Swah Tatsaviturvarenyam Bhargo Devasya Dhimahi Dhiyo Yo Naha Prachodyat**" (May Almighty illuminate our intellect and inspire us towards the righteous path) but the intellectual understanding of the meaning of mantra, although good, is not in itself sufficient to make it efficacious. It does not encompass all the variegated dimensions of a mantra.

A mantra may have a meaning, or it may not have one. It may be sublime thought, or it may not be. Many times, the arrangement of its syllables is such as to give out a meaning, while at other times, this construction is so haphazard that no intelligible meaning can be made out of it. There are several other Mantras like:

Om Namo Bhagavate Vasudevaya,

Om Namo Narayanaya,

Hari Om,

Hari Om Tat Sat.

Maha-Mrtywijaya Mantra:

"Om Tryambakam Yajamahe Sugandhim Puitivardhanam Urvarukamiva Bandhanan Mrtyor Muldiya Mamrtat".

Om Namah Ivttya, etc.

By Mantra - Sadhana, certain secret recesses or zones of the Sadhak's interior become activated, and he becomes capable of receiving, bearing and harnessing those subtle energies. Only then the mantra is said to have become siddha (accomplished or mastered).

If everything is performed correctly, siddhi of the mantra is inevitable. Mantra siddhi means energies of the Mantra becoming active in the arena of Sadhak's inner consciousness. This condition may be roughly likened to a hard working farmer digging a long canal and bringing the waters of a great river to his fields. Just as completion of the canal leads to his whole agricultural lands being permanently irrigated and saturated with waves of water, even so, after Siddhi of the Mantra the energy flow of

Devasakti keeps gushing and pouring every moment into the inner consciousness of the Sadhak. He can employ this force according to his resolve. He can cure incurable ailments by the potency of specific mantras.

The methodology of a mantra's functioning is novel. As the specific phase of its Sadhana is completed, it connects the Sadhak's inner consciousness with the specific cosmic energy current or Deva Sakti. But this is one aspect of its function. In its other aspect, it simultaneously makes the Sadhak qualified and fit to receive this special power. By mantra- Sadhana, certain secret recesses or zones of the Sadhak's interior become activated, and he becomes capable of receiving, bearing and harnessing those subtle energies. Only then the mantra is said to have become siddha (accomplished or mastered). This Mantra Siddhi does not come by mere rote chanting or mechanical repetition. This explains why a good many persons even after years of Sadhana of a mantra have to meet with disappointment. Either they get no result at all or only partial and negligible result. The fault lies not with the mantra but with the Sadhak. It is important to bear in mind that any mantra - Sadhana requires the Sadhak to attune his life to the peculiar nature of the mantra.

Significance of Mantra Yoga

When a mantra is chanted in rhythmic tone with ups and downs, they create a melodious effect in the body. This effect can be defined as the Neuro-linguistic effect. The Neuro-linguistic effect will be possible even if you do not know the meaning of the mantra. Hence knowing the meaning of every mantra is not compulsory.

At the same time if you know the meaning it has got an additional effect which is known as Neuro-linguistic (NLE) + Psycholinguistic effect (PLE). Lot of Research studies have been carried out by many and important results derived by one of the famous professors Dr. T. Temple Tutler, of the Cleveland University, USA on these effects are remarkable. The NLE and PLE effects are due to the production and spreading of curative chemicals in the brain. These curative chemicals give smoothening and curing effect in the body. Thus mantra chanting is no way a superstition. It can also be directly called as music therapy or mantra therapy in modern words.

Listening to mantras directly lowers blood pressure, normalizes heart beat rate, brain wave pattern, adrenalin level, even cholesterol level. That is the reason why modern doctors advise the people under high tension to sit and listen to music or mantras for few minutes. This has become an accepted procedure just like the yoga and Pranayam practices. Even chanting the Kirtans, melodious Bhajans, songs, etc., have the good effect almost similar to the NLE and PLE. However there should a melodious pattern for that. The music/ song/mantra should never be hard/ harsh/rough/ etc. The speed also should have a smoothening effect for example even Gayatri mantra chanting should be done at the range of 4 - 8 numbers per minute, Om Namo Narayanaaya at 38-62 and Om Namah Sivaaya at 42-68 range per minute.[40]

Chanting the mantras every-day is excellent and important at a particular time. In physics the time, space and observer are the three important factors. Exactly like that the time, space and the person connected with chanting/listening mantras are three important factors for deriving benefit of mantras. Hence Sareera Shuddhi, Aahara Shuddhi, Mana Shuddhi, Vaak Shuddhi and Karma Shuddhi are essential for deriving the full benefit of chanting the mantra. Also the place where you are sitting should give calming effect, comfortable feeling etc. The ideal timings are the Prabhata Sandhya and Saayam Sandhya. (Morning & evening) Group chanting is excellent. Absolutely no mistake is expected in Vedic mantra chanting. When you are sick due to ill health or old age, one need not worry too much about his incapability of chanting the mantras. Mantras are chanted for solving our problems and for positive effects but mantra chanting/ not chanting should not become another problem for us. The ideal sound for mantra chanting can be maintained if possible at radius 7 meters. Veda mantras chanting is not easy so it is advised not to chant without the guidance from a Guru.[41]

---

[40] Retrieved on 04.10.2014 [http://www.yogsadhna.com]
[41] ibid www.yogsadhna.com

Other Significance:

1. Reduces Anxiety and Depression
2. Releases Neuroses
3. It is Soothing
4. Engenders Compassion
5. Boosts Immunity
6. It is Easy
7. It is Free
8. Opens Intuition
9. Increases Radiance
10. It is Empowering[42]

Mantras act upon our bodies by reprogramming the vibrations of the cells that have somehow gone askew. They restore the pattern of sounds at the heart of each and every cell, thus pushing the cells toward harmonious health.

Mantras affect not only our physical body but also our subtle body - our emotions, intellect and soul. They positively affect our aura - the energy shields surrounding our body.[43]

---

[42] Retrieved on 04.10.2014
[http://www.spiritvoyage.com/blog/index.php/10-reasons-to-chant-on-the-benefits-of-mantra-meditation/]
[43]Retrieved on 04.10.2014
[http://www.healthandyoga.com/html/news/mantra.aspx]

CHAPTER - 10

KUNDALINI YOGA

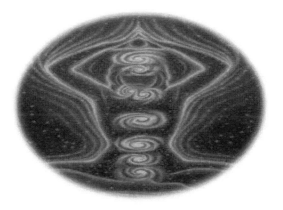

Figure No. 9 Kundalini Yoga [44]

The human body is the most excellent boon conferred by the Almighty and the person who comprehends his own body completely, realizes the subtle mysteries of the entire universe all universal faculties are concentrated as the force of life inside a human body which the scriptures term as the vital power known as Kundalini. Kundalini is derived from a Sanskrit word Kunda which means a pit. Another root is Kundal and which means the 'coiled one' basically it is the divine cosmic energy. The absolute pure energy: the power of the self which is permeating every visible and invisible reality, including the mind which grasps them. Kundalini is also symbolizes the spiritual energy that lies a serpent, at

---

[44] Retrieved on 04.10.2014
[http://www.3ho.org/files/styles/half_width/public/cosmic_chakras_-small.jpg]

the base of the spine. Every human has Kundalini: however, in most human and half circles coil.[45]

Kundalini is the power that is required to attain the ultimate goal of spiritual achievement, the union with divine (yoga) when the aspirant emerges successful in his endeavour, he gets divine vision and visualizes his real form though his divine eye, he feels overwhelmed with ecstasy and thus liberates himself from the corporeal bondages of life and death. Super sensual visions appear before the mental eve of the aspirant new worlds with indescribable wonders and charms unfold themselves before the yogi, planes after ;lanes reveal their existence and grandeur to the practitioner and the yogi gets divine knowledge, power and bless, in increasing degrees, when Kundalini passes through Chakra after Chakra, making them to bloom in all their glory which before the touch of Kundalini do not give out their powers, emanating their divine light and fragrance and reveal the divine secrets and phenomena which lie concealed form the eyes of worldly-minded people who would refuse to believe of their existence even.

According to the Philosophy of Tantra, the entire universe is a manifestation of pure consciousness, in manifesting the universe this pure consciousness seems to become divided into two poles or aspects, neither of which can exist without the other one aspect, siva, is masculine, retains a static quality and remains to be but not the power to become or change. The other aspect great mother of the

---

[45] K. Kumar; (2009), *Super Science of Yoga*, p.p. 166-174, Standard Publishers (India) New Delhi

universe for it is from her that all form is born. According to Tantra, the human being is a miniature universe. All that is found in the cosmos can be found within each individual and the same principles that apply to the universe apply in the case of the individual being. In human beings, Sakti, the feminine aspect is called Kundalini. This potential energy is said to rest at the base of the spinal cord. The object of the tantric practice of Kundalini-yoga is to awaken this cosmic energy and make it ascend through the psychic centres the chakras, which lie along the axis of the spine as consciousness potentials. She will then unite above the crown of the head with Siva the pure consciousness. This union is the aim of Kundalini-yoga: a resolution of duality into unity again a fusion with the absolute by this union the adept attains liberation while living which is considered in yogic terms to be the highest experience : a union of the individual with the universe.

Kundalini –experience are often understood in terms of the yogic chakra system. The psycho-spiritual energy centres along the spine. According to yogic tradition the Kudalini rises from the root chakra up through the spinal channel. Called susumna, and it is believed to activate each chakra it goes through. Each chakra is said to contain special characteristics. In raising Kundalini, spiritual powers (siddhis) are also believed to arise.

To understand the process it will be relevant to discuss the different psychic centres and the path through which Kundalini passes. Inside the vertebral column, there are seven subtle centers which are visualized in the form of lotus by our seers, known as chakra. Each center or lotus possesses different number of petals and also a distinct colour. The first chakra is Muladhar Chakra; this chakra is situated in the basal region of the vertebral column at the mid spot between anus and testis. During the practice of Kundalini Yoga we start with this chakra. It is visualized as a red lotus possessing four petals. This is the resting place of the Kundalini Sakti, which lies here as a snake having three and half coil. This chakra is the symbol of earth element. Activation of this chakra results in riddance from tensions, true happiness beauty, perfect health and physical strength, magnetic personality.

The second is Swadhisthan Chakra this Chakra is located in the vertebral column just opposite to the perennial region. In Kundalini yoga practice this Chakra is visualized as a vermilion coloured lotus having six petals. This semi lunar chakra is the symbol of water element. Activation of this chakra results in freedom from stomach ailments increase in sex power and cure of sexual debility, increase in courage in courage and fearlessness and magnetism.

In this system the Third Chakra is Manipur Chakra inside the vertebral column this chakra is situated just opposite to the naval region. This ten petal lotus is of blue colour. The Yantra of this chakra is triangular in shape and it represents the fire element. Activation of this chakra results in perfect digestion, riddance from ailments like kidney stones, diabetes, liver problems etc. Success in amazing Sadhanas is like flying in the air, walking on water, telepathic contact with animals and plants. Perfection in pranayama is the highest achievement.

During the practice of Kundalini yoga, the fourth chakra is Anahat Chakra, the relative position of this chakra inside the vertebral column is just opposite to the cardiac region heart. This red coloured lotus possesses twelve petals and it represents the air element. Activation of this chakra illuminates the entire body and the entire vertebral column starts vibrating. Activation of this chakra results in peace of mind, boundless divine joy, Open hearted personality, love with all, entering into Samadhi (divine trance), riddance from problems related to heart, increase in soft emotions.

The fifth step of Kundalini yoga is Visuddhi Chakra. Inside the vertebral column this chakra is located opposite the throat region. This lotus of smoky color possesses sixteen and it represents the sky element. Activation of this chakra results in riddance from all ailments related to throat, thyroid etc. Increase in knowledge, gain of power of eloquence, deeper Samadhi, perfection in the art of hypnotism, gain of power to die when one wills, total material success like comforts, Wealth, fame etc.

The sixth step in Kundalini yoga and the Master Chakra is Ajna Chakra; This Chakra is located just opposite the mid spot between the two eyebrows. This white lotus has only two petals, also called the third eye. Its activation brings wondrous powers like clairvoyance, telepathy, power of giving curses or blessing, instant fulfilment of anything one wishes and gain of knowledge related to all subjects and sciences, power to control thoughts of others and interfere even in nature.

The final stage in Kundalini yoga is the highest and the last Chakra Sahasrar Chakra. Beyond these six chakras at the upper termination of the spinal cord, is the thousand petal lotus: the abode of lord Siva (Supreme Being). When the Kundalini Sakti unites itself with the Supreme Being, the aspirant gets engrossed in deep meditation during which he perceives infinite bless. This is a subtle centre in the brain on activation of Sahasrara a very fine, elixir-like secretion is produced from it which permeates the whole body thus making the human forever free of all ailments. Sahasrara Chakra is situated two inches deep inside both the temporal region and three inches deep from the mid-spot between the eyebrows that is in the middle portion of cerebral hemispheres, from the throat, it is located three inches above the palate and inside the brain it is located in a small hole above the 'Maha Vivar' foramen of cerebrum.

Awakening of Sahasrara renders the aspirant liberated from corporeal bondages and attachments. He is endowed with all kinds of divine attainments including 'Asta Siddhi' and 'Nava Nidhi'. He becomes an omniscient yogi. Being emancipated from the cycles of birth and death, he certainly achieves the final beatitude. One is fully enlightened and can there envision any event going on anywhere in the universe without entering into Samadhi. All natural elements come under one's control.

Kundalini can be awakened by Pranayama, Asana and Mudras by Hatha Yogis; by concentration and training of the mind by Raja Yogis; by devotion and perfect self-surrender by Bhaktas: by analytical will by the Jnanis; by Mantras by the Tantrikas; and by the grace of Guru (Guru

Kripa) through touch, sight or mere Sankalpa. Rising of Kundalini and its union with Siva at the Sahasrara Chakra affect the state of Samadhi and Mukti. No Samadhi is possible without awakening the Kundalini.

Problems have been known to arise from Kundalini the following side effects have been noted. Problems can persists for movements, hours, days, months, year of decades. They can also reoccur. All aspirants with an active Kundalini, experience at least a few, if not many, of these side effects generally these problems begin to occur after a few months(less likely) or years (more likely) after starting a contemplative practice, but in some cases they begin very soon after starting meditation or yoga.

Practice of Kundalini yoga is not very easy, it should be known to all the aspirant that, the aspirant may get dearth, pseudo death, psychosis, pseudo psychosis, confusion, anxiety, panic attacks depression, sadness, suicidal thoughts, urges to self-mutilate homicidal urges, arrhythmia (irregular heart beat) exacerbation of prior of current mental illness, insomnia inability to hold a job inability to talk, inability to drive, sexual pains temporary blindness, and headaches.

The only authentic and an important scripture are available on Kundalini yoga is The Yoga-Kundalyopanisad. The three methods given in the Yoga-Kundalyopanisad for the control of Prana are: Mitahara, Asana and Sakti-Chalang. Kundalini can be aroused by a twofold practice. Saraswati Chalana and the restraint of Prana are the two practices.

The process, as described in the Yoga-Kudalyopaniṣad for arousing Kundalini is sixteen counts. In inhalation it goes in only for twelve counts, thus losing four counts. The Kundalini is aroused if one can inhale Prana for sixteen counts. This is done by sitting in Padmasana and when the Pana is flowing through the left nostril and lengthening inwards for four counts more.

By the whole process of the Kundalini Yoga Sadhana, the body of the yogi attains very subtle state of the spiritual consciousness. The yogi who has attained to Samadhi experiences everything as consciousness. The aspirant realizes the oneness of the macrocosm and the microcosm. Because, the Kundalini Sakti has reached the Sahasrara Kamala or the thousand petal lotus and has become united with Siva the aspirant enjoys the highest stage. This is the final beatitude.

Those aspirants, who aspire to arouse the Kundalini Sakti to enjoy the bliss of union of Siva and Sakti through awakened Kundalini and to gain the accompanying powers or Siddhis, should practice Kundalini Yoga. To them, this Yoga Kundalyopanisad is of great importance. It equips them with a comprehensive knowledge of the methods and processes of the Kundalini Yoga in which the Khechari Mudra stands prominent.

The Kundalini Yoga practitioner seeks to obtain both Bhakti and Mukti. He attains liberation in and through the world. Jnana yoga is the path of asceticism and liberation. Kundalini yoga is the path of enjoyment and liberation.

The aspirant of hatha yoga seeks a body which shall be as strong as steel, healthy, free from suffering and therefore long-lived. Master of the body the yogi is the master of life and death. His shining form enjoys the vitality of youth. He lives as long as he has the will to live and enjoys in the world of forms. His death is the death at will (lchho Mrtyu). The yogi should seek the guidance of an expert and skilled guru.

The Serpent Power is the power which is the static support or Adhara of the whole of the whole body and all its moving Pranic forces. The polarity as it exists in, and as, the body is destroyed by yoga which disturbs the equilibrium of bodily consciousness. Which consciousness is the result of the maintenance of these two poles? In the human body the potential pole of energy which is the Supreme Power stirred to action. The Sakti is moved upward to unite with the Siva the quiescent consciousness in the Sahasrara.

By Pranayama and other Yogic processes the static Sakti is affected and becomes dynamic. When completely dynamic when Kundalini unites with Siva in the Sahasrara the polarization or the body gives way. The two poles are united in one and there is the state of consciousness called Samadhi. The polarization takes place in the consciousness. The body actually continues to exist as an object of observation to others.

When the Kundalini ascends, the body of the yogi is maintained by the nectar which flow from the union of Siva and Shakti in Sahasrara. Glory to mother Kundalini who through her infinite grace and power kindly leads the Sadhaka from Chakra to Chakra and illumines him and makes him realize his identity with the Supreme Brahman! The yoga Kundalini Upanisad attaches great importance to the search for and finding of right Guru. It insists upon revering the illumined Guru as God Guru is one who has full self-illumination. He removes the veil of ignorance in the deluded individuals.

Whatever the mode of activation a Guru is a must for during the process as the divine powers in the body come to life they attack the Sadhak's weaknesses like greed jealousy, infatuation anger false ego and other negative traits. Sometimes the struggle between these positive and negative energies can be so intense that a person may lose balance of mind or his evil traits may appear so magnified to him that he may take to wrong ways in life. The yoga Kundalyopanisad gives a list of the obstacles to yoga practice. Some take to the practice of yoga and later on when they come across some obstacles in the way, they do not know how to proceed further. They do not know how to obviate them. Many are the obstacles, dangers, snares and pitfalls on the spiritual path. Sadhakas may commit many mistakes on the path. A Guru, who has already trodden the path and reached the goal, is very necessary to guide them.

Significance of Kundalini Yoga

Kundalini yoga is a form of physical and meditative yoga that comprises of various techniques using the mind, our senses and the body. The usage of these, results in a peaceful and relaxing communication between the soul and the body.

Kundalini yoga gives special consideration to the role of the spine and the endocrine system, which is an essential part for yogic awakening. It focuses on psycho-spiritual growth and the potential of the body for maturity.

The practice of kundalini yoga consists of a various bodily postures, expressive movements and utterances, characterological cultivations, breathing patterns, and degrees of concentration. Like all other forms of yoga, Kundalini also links movement with breadth. The way it differs is its direct focus on moving energy through the chakra system, stimulating the energy in the lower chakras and moving it to the higher chakras. Kundalini Yoga awakens the energy that resides in the spine.

Although Kundalini is very much a physical form of yoga, the main benefit is derived from the inner experience. Most popularly known as the 'Yoga of awareness', Kundalini yoga awakens the unlimited potential already existing in all human beings. When this energy is awakened in the body, it gives the individual enhanced intuition and mental clarity and creative potential.

It is a yoga designed for householders, for people who have to cope with the daily challenges and stressful life at work and at home, raising families, and managing businesses etc.

One interesting fact of Kundalini yoga is that Kundalini yoga is one of the few paths of yoga that allows sex. Medical research on kundalini yoga states that its regular practice can very much increase your sexual energy levels leading to a magnificently improved sex life.[46]

Kundalini yoga is claimed to be the foremost of yoga practices as it gives the pleasure of both Bhukti (enjoyment) and Mukti (liberation) in the fullest and literal sense. Yogis claim that Kundalini energy is far superior to all others. Which is why, the state of Samadhi attained thereby is considered most perfect. The degree, to which the unveiling of this consciousness is effected, depends upon the meditative power, and the extent of one's detachment from the world.

In Kundalini Yoga the creating and sustaining Sakti of the whole body is actually and truly united with Lord Siva. The Yogi goads Her to introduce him to Her Lord. The rousing of Kundalini Sakti and Her Union with Lord Siva affects the state of Samadhi (Ecstatic union) and spiritual Anubhava (experience). Kundalini Herself, when awakened by the Yogins, achieves for them the Jnana (illumination).

---

[46] Retrieved on 04.10.2014 [http://rootshunt.com/kundaliniyog.htm]

Practiced regularly, Kundalini can strengthen the nervous system, balance the glandular system, and harness the energy of the mind and emotion as well as the body. While general yoga technique focuses on exercise postures and breathing, Kundalini takes yoga concepts a step further by integrating them into everyday life activities.

Better functioning of your body: Kundalini Yoga, in combination with the right lifestyle changes, will put your digestive, nervous, lymphatic, cardiovascular, and glandular and all other systems in proper working order.

Beauty: Kundalini Yoga can transform many ordinary bodies into sleek physiques. Kundalini Yoga is one of the only exercise systems that recognize the importance of glandular balance in relation to physical and mental health. This has a direct bearing on your ability to look great and feel great.[47]

Sense of well-being: This comes as a result of the increased energy and relaxation, which Kundalini Yoga gives, and from the process of self-discovery and confidence you feel when you pay attention to your inner life.

Emotional balance: This attribute helps you to be the master of your life and not allow subjective mental states to cloud your ability to make clear decisions and act in accordance with your true values.

---

47 ibid http://rootshunt.com

Increases sensory awareness: The ability to touch, taste, feel and see with sensitivity, and to put your perceptions into the framework of knowledge you can use.

Enhances intuitive power: The sixth sense is a gift we all possess. Kundalini Yoga works on your higher brain centers, and gives you the nuance to compute the particulars of any situation and to arrive at a set of certainties you can bet on. Stronger intuition also alerts us of dangers and we do not attract negative forces.

Eliminates negative habits: Frequently we feel the need to compensate or self-destruct, due to a deep hurt or unresolved life issue. This can take the form of overeating, drinking, drugs and other indulgences. In the context of Kundalini Yoga there are specific techniques to help you get to the bottom of what is bothering you. Many negative habit patterns just fall away as a result of the applied practice of Kundalini Yoga.[48]

Creativity: Beyond artistic ability, creativity is a state of mind that allows you to be spontaneous, industrious, and expressive. Kundalini Yoga can help make any thing you do a personal statement.[49]

---

[48] ibid http://rootshunt.com
[49] ibid http://rootshunt.com

SUMMARY

Yoga is a science of right living and it work when integrated in our daily life. It works on all aspects of the person-the physical, mental, emotional, and psychic and spirituals. Generally the word 'Yoga' means 'Union'. Etymologically it has been derived from Sanskrit root 'Yuj' which means to bind, join attach or yoke.

Major branches of yoga in Hindu philosophy include Bhakti Yoga, Jnana Yoga, Karma Yoga, Raja Yoga, and Hatha Yoga, Dhyan Yoga, Mantra Yoga, Kundalini Yoga. Raja Yoga, compiled in the Yoga Sutras of Patanjali, and known simply as yoga in the context of Hindu philosophy, is part of the Samkhya tradition. Many other Hindu texts discuss aspects of yoga, including Upanishads, the Bhagavad Gita, the Hatha Yoga Pradipika, the Shiva Samhita and various Tantras.

Bhakti Yoga is the easiest and natural way for God – realization. It is deeply concerned with our life. This path of devotion is for everyone. Anybody can practice it. Even the vilest man can start and gradually improvement will take place. Bhakti Yoga is the way to balance the emotions by directing them towards Ishwar. This path appeals mainly to those of an emotional nature.

The word Jnana literary means knowledge and wisdom, thus it is known as Yoga of Knowledge and wisdom. This path of yoga deals directly with the highest of all human desires – the desire to know the Truth – and it gives an explanation of what Truth means and shows the practical way of realizing it. Jnana Yoga is a path for the devotee to experience unity with Ishwar by breaking the layer of ignorance that rests between.

Karma Yoga is defined as "discipline of action" or "performance of action with un-attachment to the result and the action itself". The Karma comes from Sanskrit root 'Kri' which means to do karma literary means action, which everyone performs in this world, whether consciously or unconsciously. The human beings have a natural tendency to perform some thing.

The word raja yoga is found in many of the Upanishads. It may be regarded as the master of all the yogic practices. All the yogic practices lead to Samadhi, but the specialty of this path is that it starts from, Samadhi. Hence the Samadhi comes in every path, thus it has been considered to be the complimentary practice of yoga or the greatest path of yoga. Raj-Yoga is also known as Ashtanga Yoga. Asht is translated to 8 & Anga is translated to part/limb. Therefore Raj Yoga is the yoga of 8 limbs. It is a royal (Raj = Royal) path to the happiness and peace. More than 2500 years ago in Bharat (India) Rishi Patanjali put this practice of YOGA into a system called Ashtanga Yoga.

The word 'Hatha' is made up of two Bija mantras: 'Ha' and 'Tha' where 'Ha' represents Sun or Pingala Nadi and 'Tha' represents Moon or Ida Nadi. Basically the union of these two Nadies is called hatha yoga. The aim of hatha yoga is to have the mastery over body and mind. The main objective is to create an absolute balance of the interacting activities and processes of the physical body, mind and energy.

Dhyan is a state of pure consciousness, which transcends the inner and outer senses. The word meditation is derived from two Latin words: Meditari (to think, to dwell upon and to exercise the mind) and Meditari (to heal). Meditation usually refers to a state in which the body is consciously relaxed and the mind is allowed to become calm and focused. The climax of Dhyana is Samadhi, in Indian tradition, it is used for inner soul illumination, and western psychologists link it with a special state of mind.

By the combination of *'Man'* and *'Tra'* comes Mantra. The root *'Man'* in the word Mantra comes from the first syllable of that word, meaning 'to think', and *'Tra'* from *'Trai'* meaning to protect' or 'free' from the bondage of *Samsara* or the phenomenal world. Mantras have great significance in the mental and spiritual evolution of harmony.

Kundalini yoga is a form of physical and meditative yoga that comprises of various techniques using the mind, our senses and the body. The usage of these, results in a peaceful and relaxing communication between the soul and the body. Kundalini is derived from a Sanskrit word Kunda which means a pit.

BIBLIOGRAPHY

BOOKS:

Bhaktivedanta Swami Prabhupada (2009), *Srimadbhagvad Gita*, Gitapress Gorakhpur, India

Harikrishnadas Goyandka (1996), *Patanjali Yoga Sutra,* Gitapress Gorakhpur, India

Kamakhya Kumar (2009), *Super Science of Yoga,* Standard Publishers (India) New Delhi

Swami Chinmayananda (2008), *Narada Bhakti Sutras*, Central ChinmayaMission Trust Mumbai, India

Swami Digambarji (1997), *Gheranda Samhita,* Kaivalyadhama S.M.Y.M. Samiti Lonavla, India

Swami Muktibodhananda (2005), *Hatha Yoga Pradipika,* Yoga Publications Trust, Munger, Bihar, India

Swami Niranjanananda Saraswati (2013), *Gheranda Samhita,* Yoga Publications Trust, Munger, Bihar, India

Swami Satyanand Saraswati (2013), *Four Chapter on Freedom*, Yoga Publications Trust, Munger, Bihar, India

WEBSITES:

[http://hinduism.about.com/od/thegita/a/gitabhakti.htm] Retrieved on 04.10.2014

[http://rootshunt.com/kundaliniyog.htm] Retrieved on 04.10.2014 [http://www.abc-of-yoga.com/beginnersguide/yogahistory.asp] Retrieved on 02.10.2014

[http://www.abc-of-yoga.com/beginnersguide/yogahistory.asp] Retrieved on 02.10.2014

[http://www.advaitayoga.org/excerpts/excerpts14.html] Retrieved on 04.10.2014

[http://www.akhandjyoti.org/?Akhand-Jyoti/2004/Sept-Oct/DhyanBenefits/] Retrieved on 04.10.2014

[http://www.brahmakumaris.org/us/massachusetts/typeb.20 09-07-23.5593975822/typec.2009-07-23.9541270677] Retrieved on 04.10.2014

[http://www.clivir.com/lessons/show/history-of-yoga-classification-of-yoga-history-into-four-periods.html] Retrieved on 04.10.2014

[http://www.ekhartyoga.com/everything-yoga/yoga-styles/hatha-yoga] Retrieved on 04.10.2014

[http://www.hathayogaillustrated.com/benefits-of-hatha-yoga/] Retrieved on 04.10.2014

[http://www.healthandyoga.com/html/news/mantra.aspx] Retrieved on 04.10.2014

[http://www.hinduism.co.za/jnana-.htm] Retrieved on 04.10.2014

[http://www.mkgandhi.org/talksongita/chap03.htm]
Retrieved on 04.10.2014

[http://www.spiritvoyage.com/blog/index.php/10-reasons-to-chant-on-the-benefits-of-mantra-meditation/] Retrieved on 04.10.2014

[http://www.swamil.com/history-yoga.htm] Retrieved on 02.10.2014

[http://www.swamil.com/history-yoga.htm] Retrieved on 02.10.2014

[http://www.venkatesaya.com/512.sutras/narada.php?p=01_02&menuid=2] Retrieved on 04.10.2014

[http://www.yogaindailylife.org/esystem/yoga/en/170300/the-four-paths-of-yoga/raja-yoga/] Retrieved on 04.10.2014

[http://www.yogamag.net/archives/1992/djuly92/bhkyog.shtml] Retrieved on 04.10.2014

[http://www.yogsadhna.com/index.php?option=com_content&view=article&id=203&Itemid=136] Retrieved on 04.10.2014

[http://yoga.ygoy.com/2010/05/22/the-history-yoga-preclassical-yoga/] Retrieved on 04.10.2014

[http://yoga108.org/pages/show/108-meditation-definition-and-benefits] Retrieved on 04.10.2014

[http://yoga108.org/pages/show/55-jnana-yoga-introduction] Retrieved on 04.10.2014

ABOUT THE AUTHOR(S)

Dr. Vineet Kumar Sharma is a former Assistant Professor at the Lovely Professional University Jalandhar. He is emerging writer in the field of Yoga and Physical Education. He has experience of more than eight years in the field of yogic practices. He did Bachelors (B.P.Ed), Masters (M.P.Ed) and Ph.D. degree in Physical Education with the specialization of Yogic Sciences from the Lakshmibai National Institute of Physical Education, Gwalior. He has written his Ph.D thesis on "Effect of Suryanamaskar with Breathing and Mantras on Selected Psycho-Physiological Variables". He has published more than 10 papers/articles to his credit in reputed journals on various yogic practices. He has also organized various yoga camps and training sessions like summer camps (LNIPE Gwalior), training camps (for national army shooter), etc.

Dr. Sunil Deshmukh is presently Yoga Instructor in Department of Yogic Sciences, LNIPE Gwalior. He has been actively associated with teaching, training and research for more than 20 years.

Printed in Great Britain
by Amazon